GW00994564

Walking for ~~~~~
and Fitness

The Easiest Way to Get in Shape and Stay in Shape

Frank S. Ring

Edition 1

April 7, 2020

Published by:

Walking for Health and Fitness
PO Box 1208
Oakland, NJ 07436
WWW.WalkingForHealthAndFitness.com

© **2020 Frank S. Ring**
All Rights Reserved

No part of this publication may be reproduced, distributed, or transmitted in any form or by any means, including photocopying, recording, or other electronic or mechanical methods, without the prior written permission of the publisher, except in the case of brief quotations embodied in critical reviews and certain other noncommercial uses permitted by copyright law.

For permission requests, write to the publisher, addressed:
"Attention: Permissions Coordinator," at the address above.

Dedication

To my son James,

You changed my life in so many incredible ways.

I walk to stay healthy so that I'll be around with you for many years to come.

Life is full of challenges and the way to overcome them is to educate yourself, take massive action, and develop confidence in your abilities.

The rewards are enormous in the growth you will experience.

Contents

About Walking for Health and Fitness

Walking for Health and Fitness is a health, fitness, and wellness website dedicated to walking and all the physical, psychological, and spiritual benefits that comes from it in order to achieve a healthy, balanced lifestyle!

Caution:
The Information contained in this book may cause you to feel better than you have ever felt in your entire life!

Symptoms Include:
A broader smile, happier disposition, brighter outlook on life, and general feelings of bliss…proceed with wild abandon!

Walk on,
Frank S. Ring

Exclusive Website Resource Page

To give you additional content, I've set a webpage designed to pass along bonus and exclusive content, and to keep in touch.

DOWNLOAD FREE BONUS CONTENT
Go To:
www.walkingforhealthandfitness.com/whf-ebook-digital-resources

- **FREE**: Audiobook Version of Walking for Health and Fitness | The Easiest Way to Get in Shape and Stay in Shape
- **FREE:** Exercise Supplemental Guide
- **FREE:** Walking Inspiration, my quarterly digital magazine.
- **FREE:** My exclusive Get Out the Door Checklist to streamline your walking and fitness routine

FREE: Additional bonus content will be added throughout the year

Program Goals

The Walking for Health and Fitness Program Goals are to assist you in:

- Developing a consistent routine in preparing to walk
- Developing good eating habits
- Developing good fitness routine habits
- Enjoying the walking lifestyle

Walking for Health and Fitness
The Easiest Way to Get in Shape and Stay in Shape!

The Walking for Health and Fitness Exercise Principles:

1. **Work to your fitness level:** increase the intensity as you get stronger
2. **Be consistent:** avoid long period of inactivity
3. Follow an effective routine
4. **Set realistic goals:** goals keep you on track
5. **Record your activities:** keeping a log of your walking miles and fitness routines will keep you motivated when you look back and see just how much you have accomplished
6. Make the plan fit your lifestyle
7. Work on your mindset
8. Short bodyweight fitness workouts (32-minutes is all you need)
9. **Get inspired: read uplifting books** and listen to audiobooks while you walk
10. **Experiment:** try different things
11. **Make the time:** you don't find time, you make the time to walk
12. **Be patient:** fitness doesn't travel on a straight line
13. **Be happy:** its better than being sad
14. **Reward yourself:** celebrate your accomplishments

Getting in shape is not difficult when you have the right mindset.

Please keep this in mind; you are exercising to get in shape in terms of your cardiovascular system and your muscle strength. Being able to walk for longer periods and increasing your muscle strength will serve you well over the long term, and by long term I mean the rest of your life!

You are not training as if you are an Olympic athlete. If you were training for the Olympics, you would have a training regime that is specific to the event you are competing in. Marathon runners train for miles and miles at a time. Sprinters run shorter, more intense workouts, followed by heavy weight training.

You are training for your own Olympics, the Olympics of the rest of your life. You'll need to be mobile well into advanced age, strong enough to get you to that old age, and most important, if you enjoy the fitness walking process, then it's a win-win.

While all the marathon runners, basketball players, and Boot-camp/Cross-fit devotes are dealing with knee and hip replacement, **you will be walking on!**

Introduction

I have good news for you: good health and fitness just became easy!

I promise you that a month from now, you will feel better than you do today!

There are many ways to get yourself in shape, but walking will give you the most "bang for the buck"!

> *You've just stepped into your home; a healthy glow lights*
> *up your face as you've just walked for 30 minutes straight.*
> *The scent of the crisp fresh morning air follows you into*
> *your living room. You feel reinvigorated and more alive*
> *than you have in years; Who knew walking could have such*
> *a powerful impact on your life?*

"If it's to be, it's up to me".
–Dr. Dennis Waitley

Walking is gentle on the body and soothing to the mind. Walking allows you to experience the physical sensation of movement and the mind-expanding feeling that comes through physical activity.

Why the Sedentary Lifestyle is Dangerous
By definition, the sedentary lifestyle is characterized by spending a majority of your time sitting or lying down with little or no exercise. Some experts consider this as dangerous as smoking.

We sit when we eat breakfast, sit for the morning commute, most of us sit at a desk all day, sit for lunch, sit for the evening commute, sit for dinner, sit for television or computer time.

Then, we end our day by lying down and sleeping for 6 to 8 hours every evening.

11

What You Can Do to Improve Your Health and Fitness
Walking is by far the easiest and most effective way to take care of your health. A daily 30-minute walk will improve your cardiovascular health, reduce excess body fat, strengthen bones, and enhance muscle performance!

> *The doctor glances at your medical chart; looks up at you, then quickly back to the chart. "How can this be? I don't know what you're doing but the results are amazing. Let's cut your blood pressure medication in half and retest you in 6 months!"*

For people who may be predisposed to certain health conditions, walking can reduce the risk of heart disease, cancer, diabetes, arthritis, osteoporosis, back issues, Alzheimer's disease, and other dementias.

Walking is also an antidote for being overweight and obese. These conditions are known to increase blood pressure, and high blood pressure is the leading cause of strokes.

Excess weight also increases your chances of developing other problems linked to strokes, including high cholesterol, high blood sugar, and heart disease.

Obesity is one of the biggest drivers of preventable chronic diseases and healthcare costs in the United States. Currently, estimates for these costs range from $147 billion to nearly $210 billion per year.

In addition, obesity is associated with job absenteeism, costing approximately $4.3 billion annually.

Obesity causes lower productivity while at work, costing employers $506 per obese worker per year.

An Investment in Yourself!
Doctor's visits, prescriptions, lost time at work and the lessened quality of life due to preventable illness all add up to a significant sum of time and money.

As you go through this program, look at your time and effort as **an investment in yourself.**

Let me repeat that: As you go through this program, look at your time and effort as **an investment in yourself!**

What could be better than that? Your health, happiness, and life depend on it!

Your Next Step:
Closing Thoughts for this Chapter

- The sedentary lifestyle is dangerous.
- Walking will enhance your life in so many ways.
- Walking will ignite in you a true sense of wellbeing, which is a really wonderful feeling and is so easy to achieve.
- We will set up your program so you can enjoy the benefits forever!
- Walking is by far the easiest and most effective way to take care of your health.
- As you go through this book, look at your time and effort as an investment in yourself.

I. Getting Started

We kick off the book with the basics of getting started:

- ***Don't Become a Statistic*** will reveal the costs of not being in good health.
- ***Benefits of Walking*** will show you how walking will help you minimize the cost to your health and your wallet.
- ***Personal Goals*** will encourage you to set two goals for yourself, one will be a long-term goal, the other a short term goal.
- ***Basic Gear*** will give you the rundown on what type of shoes and clothing will make your walking experience a more positive one.
- Lastly, we bring the section to a close with the *7 **Ways Sitting Can Kill You.***

Let's begin by putting one foot in front of the other!

Chapter 1: Don't Become a Statistic

If the Walking for Health and Fitness program saves you from having to make just one trip to the doctor this year, it will more than pay back the cost of this eBook and the related Walking for Health and Fitness Complete Program.

Let me repeat that… if the Walking for Health and Fitness program saves you from having to make just one trip to the doctor this year, it will more than pay back the cost of this program!

Studies published in both the Journal of the American Heart Association and The Lancet concluded that a person who exercises five times per week paid $2,500 less in annual health care expenses related to heart disease than someone who did not walk or otherwise move for 30 minutes per day, five times per week!

As you'll later see, the cost of most preventable diseases is staggering.

Doctor's visits, prescriptions, lost time at work, and the lost quality of life due to preventable illness all add up to a significant sum of time and money.

So as you go through this book, look at your time and effort as an investment in yourself. What could be better than that? Your health, happiness, and life depend on it!

Walking Speed Predicts Life Expectancy of Older Adults
Walking speed* is a powerful indicator of vitality:
Walking speed studies shows that an older person's pace, along with their age and gender, can predict their life expectancy just as well as the complex battery of other health indicators, such as blood pressure, body mass index, chronic conditions, and smoking history.

The analysis published in The Journal of the American Medical Association (JAMA), found that walking speed turned out to be a consistent predictor of survival length across age, race, and height categories, but it was especially useful in zeroing in on life expectancy for those who still live and get around independently as well as those older than 75.

Based on these studies, it's important to track a person's walking speed over time.

By tracking your walking speed, you will be more aware of hidden health problems if you suddenly start to slow down your pace.

If you feel well, yet you've slowed down, then there may be an underlying problem.

The quicker you get it resolved, the less time-consuming and expensive the treatment will be.

*The complete *Walking for Health and Fitness Program* has worksheets and instructions on how to track your walking speed over time.
For more information go to:
www.walkingforhealthandfitness.com/the-walking-program

Cost of Heart Disease:
Key Facts
Together, heart disease and stroke are among the most widespread and costly health problems facing the nation today. On a personal level, families who experience heart disease or stroke have to deal with not only medical bills, but also lost wages and the real potential of a decreased standard of living.

- Heart disease and stroke cost America nearly $1 billion a day in medical costs and lost productivity.
- Heart disease and stroke cost the nation an estimated $316.6 billion in health care costs and lost productivity in 2016.
- Approximately 1.5 million heart attacks and strokes occur every year in the United States.

- More than 800,000 people in the United States die from cardiovascular disease each year—that's 1 in every 3 deaths, and about 160,000 of them occur in people under age 65.
- Heart disease kills roughly the same number of people in the United States each year as cancer, lower respiratory diseases (including pneumonia), and accidents combined.
- Cardiovascular disease is largely preventable!

Cost of Cancer
- For patients and their families, the costs associated with direct cancer care are staggering.
- In 2014, cancer patients paid nearly $4 billion out-of-pocket for cancer treatments.
- Cancer also represents a significant proportion of total U.S. health care spending.
- Roughly $87.8 billion was spent in 2014 in the U.S. on cancer-related health care.
- Employers, insurance companies, and taxpayer-funded public programs like Medicare and Medicaid, as well as cancer patients and their families, paid these costs.

Cost of Diabetes:
- People with diagnosed diabetes incur average medical expenditures of about $13,700 per year, of which about $7,900 is attributed to diabetes.
- People with diagnosed diabetes, on average, have medical expenditures approximately 2.3 times higher than what expenditures would be in the absence of diabetes.

Cost of Being Overweight
- Overweight and obesity are known to increase blood pressure.
- High blood pressure is the leading cause of strokes.
- Excess weight also increases your chances of developing other problems linked to strokes, including high cholesterol, high blood sugar, and heart disease.

- Obesity is one of the biggest drivers of preventable chronic diseases and healthcare costs in the United States.
- Currently, estimates for these costs range from $147 billion to nearly $210 billion per year.
- In addition, obesity is associated with job absenteeism, costing approximately $4.3 billion annually.
- Obesity causes lower productivity while at work, costing employers $506 per obese worker per year.

Health Care Costs Steadily Increase With Body Mass
Researchers at Duke Medicine are giving people another reason to lose weight in the New Year: obesity-related illnesses are expensive.

According to a study published in the journal Obesity, health care cost increases parallel body mass measurements, even beginning at a recommended healthy weight.

The researchers found that costs associated with medical and drug claims rose gradually with each unit increase in body mass index (BMI). Notably, these increases began above a BMI of 19, which falls in the lower range of the healthy BMI category.

"Our findings suggest that excess fat is detrimental at any level," said lead author Truls Østbye, M.D., Ph.D., professor of community and family medicine at Duke and Professor of Health Services and Systems Research at Duke-National University of Singapore.

While this is a community-based study, think about how much money you have saved by walking… $5.60 for every $1 invested! That's a return on investment that Warren Buffet wouldn't pass on!

A 2008 study by the Urban Institute, The New York Academy of Medicine and TFAH found that an investment of $10 per person in proven community-based programs to increase physical activity, improve nutrition, and prevent smoking and other tobacco use could save the country more than $16 billion annually within five years.

That's a return of $5.60 for every $1 invested!

Out of the $16 billion, Medicare could save more than $5 billion and Medicaid could save more than $1.9 billion. Also, expanding the use of prevention programs would better inform the most effective, strategic public and private investments that yield the strongest results.

Cost of Back Pain
Low back pain (LBP) has a major economic impact in the United States, with total costs related to this condition exceeding $100 billion per year(Journal of the American Osteopathic Association).

An analysis by the Journal of the American Medical Association (JAMA) on health care spending in the United States revealed that low back and neck pain accounted for the third highest amount of spending at $87.6 billion (US Spending on Personal Health Care and Public Health, 1996-2013, December 27, 2016).

Cost of Back Pain and Related Issues
The cost of treatment for patients with low back pain (LBP) has a major economic impact worldwide. In the United States, patients with musculoskeletal conditions incur total annual medical care costs of approximately $240 billion, of which $77 billion is related to musculoskeletal conditions.

According to a 2006 review, total costs associated with LBP in the United States exceed $100 billion per year, two-thirds of which are a result of lost wages and reduced productivity.

How Walking Benefits Back Pain Sufferers

Walking is a much lower-impact activity than running. Most back pain is relieved with walking, and you can enjoy other great benefits as well.

By adopting a regular walking routine, you will strengthen your hips, legs, ankles, and feet, as well as your core.
This helps to provide better stability for your spine. It also helps to increase circulation in the spinal structures, draining toxins, and pumping nutrients into the surrounding soft tissues.

Pain often restricts mobility. Walking helps to improve range of motion and flexibility. You will find that your posture improves as well as your mood.

A stronger body and increased flexibility help to prevent injury.

Walking at least three times a week for at least 30 minutes is great for overall wellness and a strong body. Combine it with a healthy diet and stress relief techniques, and you will look, feel, and move better, and your pain will be easier to manage.

Cost of Arthritis

The total costs for arthritis in the U.S. may exceed 2% of the country's gross domestic product!

Arthritis is the leading cause of disability in the United States, limiting everyday activities for more than 7 million Americans.

In many cases, arthritis deprives individuals of their independence and disrupts the lives of family members and other caregivers.

In addition, disabilities from arthritis create enormous costs for individuals, their families, and the nation.

Each year, arthritis results in 44 million outpatient visits and almost three-quarters of a million hospitalizations.

Estimated medical care costs for people with arthritis are $15 billion annually, and total costs (medical care and lost productivity) are estimated at almost $65 billion annually.

Walking helps ease the effects of arthritis as it increases strength and flexibility, reduces joint pain, and helps combat fatigue.

Cost of Alzheimer's and Other Dementias
In 2017, the cost to the nation will be $259 billion dollars.
35% of caregivers for people with Alzheimer's and other dementias reported that their health has gotten worse due to the responsibilities of providing care.

Please take note: 1 in 3 seniors dies with Alzheimer's or other forms of dementia.

Regular physical activity has many benefits for people with Alzheimer's disease.

Exercise helps keep muscles, joints, and the heart in good shape. It also helps people stay at a healthy weight and can improve sleep.

"Nothing tastes as good as fit feels"

Your Next Step:
You must decide right now not to become a statistic. You have it within yourself to take control of your health!

Do not waste another second in ill health. Take a break from reading and get out and walk somewhere right now!

Even a stroll around the block will get you moving in the right direction.

Chapter 2: Benefits of Walking

Why am I so enthusiastic about walking? Well, I'll give you 3 reasons: its free, it's easy to do, and it's easy on your body's muscles, joints, and bones!

There's no question that walking is good for you. Walking is an aerobic exercise, which stimulates and strengthens the heart and lungs, thereby improving the body's utilization of oxygen.

A University of Tennessee study found that women who walked had less body fat than those who didn't walk.

It also lowers the risk of blood clots as the calf acts as a venous pump, contracting and pumping blood from the feet and legs back to the heart, reducing the load on the heart.

Walking Prevents Heart Disease
Walking is a form of aerobic exercise and is one of the easiest ways to increase your physical activity and improve your health. Exercise also increases your lungs' ability to take in oxygen, lowers blood pressure, helps to reduce body fat, and improves blood sugar and cholesterol levels.

Walking Prevents Cancer
Exercise has a number of biological effects on the body, some of which have been proposed to explain associations with specific cancers, including lowering the levels of hormones, such as insulin and estrogen, and of certain growth factors that have been associated with cancer development and progression.

Walking Prevents Obesity
Walking helps to prevent obesity and decrease the harmful effects of obesity, particularly the development of insulin resistance (failure of the body's cells to respond to insulin) by reducing inflammation and improving immune system function

Exercise, in general, alters the metabolism of bile acids, resulting in decreased exposure of the gastrointestinal tract to these suspected carcinogens thus limiting the amount of time it takes for food to travel through the digestive system, which decreases gastrointestinal tract exposure to possible carcinogens.

Walking Prevents Diabetes
One possible reason why: when you perform a moderate exercise—like walking three miles—your body taps into its stores of fatty acids to fuel it more than it does when you exercise vigorously, like if you jogged the same distance. That's good news for your diabetes risk as an elevated level of free fatty acids can make it harder for your body to process the hormone insulin.

- **Type 2 Diabetes:** A 2012 study of 201 people with type 2 diabetes found that every additional 2,600 steps (approximately 1 mile) of walking each day was associated with a 0.2% lower A1c.

- **Pre-diabetes/Overweight/Obese:** A 2007 analysis, which included five studies examining walking and the risk of type 2 diabetes (data from a staggering 301,221 people), found that those who walked regularly—about 20 minutes per day— had a 30% lower risk of developing type 2 diabetes.

Walking Helps Improve Back Pain
Walking is a much lower impact activity than running. Most back pain is relieved with walking and you can enjoy other great benefits as well. By adopting a regular walking routine, you will strengthen your hips, legs, ankles, and feet, as well as your core.

This helps to provide better stability for your spine. It also helps to increase circulation in the spinal structures, draining toxins, and pumping nutrients into the surrounding soft tissues.

Pain often restricts mobility. Walking helps to improve range of motion and flexibility. You will find that your posture improves as well as your mood. A stronger body and increased flexibility help to prevent injury.

Walking at least three times a week for at least 30-minutes is great for overall wellness and a strong body.

Combine it with a healthy diet and stress relief techniques and you will look, feel, and move better – and your pain will be easier to manage.

Walking Improves Circulation
It also wards off heart disease, brings up the heart rate, lowers blood pressure and strengthens the heart. Women who walked 30 minutes a day reduced their risk of stroke by 20 percent, and by 40 percent when they stepped up the pace, according to researchers at the Harvard School of Public Health in Boston.

Studies at the University of Colorado at Boulder and the University of Tennessee found that post-menopausal women who walked just one to two miles a day lowered blood pressure by nearly 11 points in 24 weeks.

Walking Stops the Loss of Bone Mass
Walking can stop the loss of bone mass for those with osteoporosis, according to Michael A. Schwartz, MD, of Plancher Orthopedics & Sports Medicine in New York.

Walking Lightens the Mood
A California State University, Long Beach, study showed that the more steps people took during the day, the better their moods were. Why? Walking releases natural pain-killing endorphins to the body, one of the emotional benefits of exercise.

Walking Leads to Weight Loss
A quick 30-minute walk burns 200 calories. Over time, calories burned can lead to pounds dropped.

Walking Strengthens Muscles
Walking tones your leg and abdominal muscles– and even arm muscles—
if you pump them as you walk. This increases your range of motion,
shifting the pressure and weight away from your joints and muscles, which
are meant to handle the weight, helping to lessen arthritis pain.

**A Brigham and Women's Hospital, Boston, study of post-menopausal
women found that 30 minutes of walking each day reduced their risk
of hip fractures by 40 percent.**

Walking Improves Sleep
A study from the Fred Hutchinson Cancer Research Center in Seattle
found that women, ages 50 to 75, who took one-hour morning walks, were
more likely to relieve insomnia than women who didn't walk.

Walking Supports Your Joints
The majority of joint cartilage has no direct blood supply. It gets its
nutrition from the synovial or joint fluid that circulates as we move. The
impact that comes from movement or compression, such as walking,
"squishes" the cartilage, bringing oxygen and nutrients into the area. If
you don't walk, joints are deprived of life-giving fluid, which can speed
deterioration.

Walking Improves Your Breath
When walking, your breathing rate increases, causing oxygen to travel
faster through the bloodstream, helping to eliminate waste products and
improve your energy level and the ability to heal.

Walking Slows Mental Decline
A study of 6,000 women, ages 65 and older, performed by researchers at
the University of California, San Francisco, found that age-related
memory decline was lower in those who walked more. The women
walking 2.5 miles per day had a 17-percent decline in memory, as opposed
to a 25-percent decline in women who walked less than a half-mile per
week.

25

Walking Lowers Alzheimer's Risk
A study from the University of Virginia Health System in Charlottesville found that men between the ages of 71 and 93 who walked more than a quarter of a mile per day had half the incidence of dementia and Alzheimer's disease, compared to those who walked less.

Walking Helps You Do More, Longer
Aerobic walking and resistance exercise programs may reduce the incidence of disability in the daily activities of people who are older than 65 and have symptomatic OA, shows a study published in the Journal of Clinical Outcomes Management.

Walking Leads to a Longer Life
Research out of the University of Michigan Medical School and the Veterans Administration Ann Arbor Healthcare System says those who exercise regularly in their fifties and sixties are 35 percent less likely to die over the next eight years than their non-walking counterparts.

That number shoots up to 45 percent less likely for those who have underlying health conditions.

Your Next Step:
If you didn't walk after the last chapter then **DO IT NOW!**

Chapter 3: Personal Goals

The late great Beatle, George Harrison, sang it best: "If you don't know where you're going, any road will take you there!"

Developing a fitness routine is a major undertaking, and having a destination to get to will keep you on track to reach the health and fitness level you'd like to achieve.

If you were looking to purchase a fancy new watch, you wouldn't get into your car and drive aimlessly around town in hopes that you'd eventually find the fancy new watch store, would you?

Without a specific destination in mind, you might wind up at a discount department store that only sells cheap watches. That's not for you!

My goal is to get you to the fancy new watch store. Or, better yet, into good health and fitness habits!

The goal setting process is the defining component of your walking program! This is why we will spend so much time on it.

Is it a Goal or a Wish?
Most people think that having a vague idea of what they want and being positive and optimistic about accomplishing it is a goal. This isn't for you!

Only 3 percent of people have clear, written goals with plans to accomplish them. Only 3 percent of people work on their most important goals each day.

You want to be among the 3 percent!

Goal Setting Made Simple
Before you actually "walk" to your goal, you need to take a series of planning steps to dramatically increase the chances that you will be successful.

These Seven Steps Will Help You to Set Your Goals!
1. Decide exactly what you want in terms of health and fitness.
2. Write down your goals and make them measurable.
3. Set a deadline.
4. Identify all the obstacles that you will have to overcome to achieve your goals.
5. Determine the additional knowledge and skills that you will require to achieve your goals.
6. Determine those people whose help and cooperation you will require to achieve your goals.
7. Make a list of all your answers to the above, and organize them by sequence and priority.

By following these seven steps, you can accomplish any goal that you set for yourself.

Your Next Step:
- Set 2 goals for yourself:
- Set one big long-term goal.
- Give yourself a compelling reason to get up and walk each day.
- Set one small goal that you can accomplish today!

We all need a win every day!

Included in the **Walking for Health and Fitness Complete Program**: Videos, simple formula, and worksheet that will guide you through the process of determining your most important destination and your number one goal!

www.walkingforhealthandfitness.com/the-walking-program

Chapter 4: Basic Gear

Walking requires little more than a good footwear—walking shoes or sneakers, some comfortable clothes, socks, and… that's it!

Footwear
To get started quickly, you just need a comfortable pair of sneakers! With that said, going forward as your walking increases, an investment in walking shoes will enhance the walking experience.

Just to be clear, you don't need any special walking shoe to start! Just wear a pair of sneakers that are comfortable.

The main goal at this point is to just get moving.

Why Walking Shoes?
Let's take a look at walking and running and the body mechanics involved with each.

As you walk, the body's weight is distributed more evenly on the foot than when you run.

When walking, your weight rolls from the heel through the ball and continues to the toe in one foot after the other. This gentler, rocking chair-like motion requires your feet to absorb the shock of only 1-2x your body weight with each step. And, during walking there are points where both feet are firmly on the ground, dividing weight.

With each walking step, the outer heel absorbs most of the impact before distributing weight through the foot in an S motion through the push-off from the toe.

In contrast, running requires the support of at least 2-3x your body weight and each stride has moments with neither foot on the ground. Runners spend a good deal of time "in the air" literally.

What Goes Up Must Come Down!
It is this constant landing that pounds and puts a tremendous amount of stress on the body over time, causing it to break down!

So What's This Mean To Your Shoes?
Basically, it's the old axiom of having the right tool for the job. Walking shoes are designed with the specific body mechanics and stride path of walking in mind.

They are constructed to be more flexible through the ball of the foot to allow a greater range of motion through the "roll" of the forefoot. They also have greater arch support to protect where the force is heaviest on the foot.

Running shoes, in contrast, have more cushioning in the heel–the point of impact–and less protection through the ball of the foot.

The amount of heat generated in the running motion is greater, so running shoes also are made with a higher amount of mesh to keep feet cool during exercise.

Picking the proper shoes can prevent discomfort, injury, and will encourage you to maintain an active lifestyle. It is most important that your shoes feel comfortable so that you do not avoid exercising.

Shoe Buying Tips
- When you shop for shoes, wear the socks you exercise in.
- The shoes should be comfortable as soon as you put them on.
- The heel ought to fit snugly, not slip up out of the shoe.
- If the shoes are tight, do not expect them to stretch out, even if they look stylish. Since feet swell during the day, shop for shoes in the afternoon or after a long walk.
- To prevent painful blisters, calluses, and to avoid foot disorders like bunions and hammertoes, check for enough room on the sides of your feet, above your toes, and about a half-inch between the end of your longest toe and the shoe.

Walking shoes that are more structured will give you stability. Look for shoes with medial (inside) support to limit over-pronation and support your feet.

Once your shoes are worn out, they must be replaced.

If you can see through the outer sole to the midsole, or feel the support buckling as you exercise, it is time for a new pair.

Even well-made shoes eventually degrade.
The best advice is to keep track of the mileage on your shoe.

On average, shoes last roughly 300-500 miles, so if you walk for exercise, keeping a weekly log of miles will help you understand when your shoes are ready to be replaced.

The best way to ensure that you will enjoy exercising is to have gear that fits right.

Where to Buy Walking Shoes
Find a local shoe store, running store, or department store.

You will get the best service, information, and fit at the shoe or running stores as the sales reps are trained in fitting your foot type. Keep in mind that in a department store, you're on your own.

Take your time, try on several pairs, and make sure they are totally comfortable. Wear the type of socks you will be wearing while walking.

Walk around the store wearing the shoe, as you will be spending a great deal of time wearing them when you begin your walking routine.

Shop for shoes later in the day, as your feet can swell up to a half- size larger during the course of the day.

When you find a pair that you love, try them out for a few days then go back and buy another pair. Shoe companies often "upgrade" the shoe models and if they discontinue the ones you love, you'll have to start the process all over again the next time you need shoes.

The old saying is true when purchasing footwear…you get what you pay for.

Socks
A good pairs of socks will absorb sweat and prevent friction between your feet and the inside of the shoe.

Test out several pairs, you want thick but not too thick. Synthetic materials like polyester, acrylic, and nylon are your best bet because they help wick away moisture and prevent blisters.

Make sure they don't bunch around the toes or gather at the heels, which can cause blisters and hot spots.

Clothing
Many pleasure walkers walk in regular clothes and this works just fine. Comfortable, nonrestrictive clothing works best!

Dress For the Weather
This is your major concern when dressing for walking. Being comfortable will keep you walking.

Dressing For Warm Weather
- Light loose top
- Shorts or short tights
- Synthetic clothing (helps moisture escape and evaporate to make you more comfortable)
- Hat, sunglasses, and sunscreen

Dressing for Cool Weather
Upper body—dress in layers
- 3 layers work better on the upper part of your body.
- Each layer acts as an insulator and traps body heat.
- I wear a thin synthetic layer followed by a heavier long sleeve shirt then an outer layer which is usually a windbreaker type of jacket or a lined jacket if it's really cold (less than 30 degrees).

Bottoms
- 1 layer is generally all you need.
- I usually wear a sweat-pant type of bottom.

Accessories
- Hat
- Gloves or mittens (mittens keep your hands warmer)
- A scarf or some other type of garment to keep the wind off your neck. I use a bandana as a scarf.
- Sunglasses on bright days and days when snow is on the ground.
- Any type of reflective gear is good to wear any time of day. The more visible you are, the safer you will be (more safety tips in a later chapter).

Dressing Rule of Thumb
- Dress for 10 degrees warmer than the outdoor temperature.
- Your body will warm up as you walk and you don't want to overheat.

Carryalls
- Fanny pack with water bottle holder
- These are very comfortable and allow your arms and hands to swing freely.
- Water
- Always carry water, even on cool days.
- Keys
- Phone
- Money

- Identification
- Emergency contact information

Reflective Gear
Reflective gear and a good flashlight/headlamp is a must when walking in the dark!

Your Next Step:
Evaluate your "walking" footwear and clothing. Again, you need nothing special to get moving, but a good quality pair of sneaker will greatly enhance the experience and make walking easier on your feet.

Chapter 5: 7 Ways Sitting Can Kill You

1. Sitting Linked to Weight Gain and Metabolic Syndrome

Too little physical activity results in weight gain. Externally, we notice our clothes fit tighter and the extra pounds tend to show up around the midsection. This is the start of the downward health cycle.

There are two types of fat that lead to unwanted weight gain.

Subcutaneous fat is the flab you can easily grasp with your hands, also known as "muffin top."

The second type is called visceral fat, which cannot be seen and is located deep within the abdominal cavity.

Visceral fat coats internal organs and has been linked to various metabolic disturbances and increases the risk of cardiovascular disease and type 2-diabetes. In women, this fat is linked to breast cancer.

Of the two, subcutaneous, or muffin top fat, while unsightly and hard to get rid of, is the least dangerous.

Visceral fat is the dangerous fat and needs to be addressed in order to keep your health from deteriorating.

Both are a direct result of a sedentary lifestyle.

2. Sitting Linked to Chronic Diseases

The number of chronic diseases also increases in direct proportion to the duration of sitting time. The problem caused by such inactivity is that sitting stops the circulation of lipase.

Lipase is an enzyme that absorbs fat and assists in the breakdown of dietary fats into smaller molecules called fatty acids and glycerol. With lipase inertia, fat does not get burned by muscles readily, but recirculates back into the bloodstream.

This inactivity further assists in storing fat deposits as body fat, which can eventually lead to clogging arteries and triggering various diseases.

On the other hand, even the simplest of activities such as standing up as opposed to sitting involves muscle participation and assists the body's ability to process cholesterol and fat in a positive manner.

Cardiovascular Disease
- The term 'cardiovascular disease' is applied to long-term conditions in which the heart cannot effectively pump blood throughout the body.
- The risk is increased manifold when individuals also maintain a sedentary lifestyle at the same time.

Type 2-Diabetes
- Sitting for long periods can elevate blood glucose levels.

Cancer
- The American Institute for Cancer Research presented estimates of 49,000 cases of breast cancer and 43,000 cases of colon cancer to be linked to a lack of physical activity.

3. Sitting Linked to Musculoskeletal Issues

A lot of muscle and bone degeneration can happen when a person sits for a long time. For instance, you may start to suffer from weak abs if you keep sitting for a long time during the day. The seated position also puts huge stress on the back muscles, neck, and spine.

The resulting tight muscles and flabby abs from bad posture can damage the spine's natural arch and lead to a condition known as hyperlordosis or swayback.

Flexible hips can help maintain balance when sitting, but incessant sitters hardly ever stretch the hip flexors and they become tight and short. This results in limiting the individual's stride length and range of motion. Plus, reduced hip mobility can then easily become a primary reason for falls in advanced age.

So while muscles suffer in one sense, bones do so in another. When people keep themselves seated for a long time, bones also become inactive.

Inactivity can cause bones to become soft and lead to serious conditions like osteoporosis.

Throw in poor or slowed circulation from prolonged sitting, and it results in fluid collecting in the legs.

The problems of impaired circulation can result in swollen ankles, varicose veins and deep vein thrombosis, to name a few. Of these, varicose veins are enlarged veins and can cause aching, pain, and discomfort for some people.

In the least severe cases, this does not present a problem, but prolonged cases of varicose veins may indicate a higher risk of other circulatory problems.

Deep vein thrombosis (DVT) is a clot that forms in the leg, often because people sit still for too long. It can be serious if the clot breaks free and lodges in the lung. Some people might notice swelling and pain, but others have no symptoms at all.

4. Sitting Linked to Brain Drain

Muscles in motion pump oxygen and blood to the brain. Sitting restricts this flow, leading to a host of neurological problems:
Anxiety and depression

There is a link between a sedentary lifestyle and the onset of anxiety and depression.

Disruption of sleep patterns
- Leading to social withdrawal and poor metabolic health.
- Brain fog also is linked to a sedentary lifestyle.

5 Sitting Linked to Organ Damage
Internal organs are greatly affected by sitting for too long.

Heart
Fatty acids lead to clogged arteries which lead to cardiovascular disease.

Pancreas
The pancreas produces insulin which carries glucose to the cells for energy. In a sedentary state, the cells in idle muscles do not respond as readily to insulin. This results in the pancreas producing too much insulin and becoming a precursor to diabetes.

Kidney
Sitting for prolonged periods of time elevate the risk factor for chronic kidney disease, particularly in women.

6. Sitting Linked to Increased Mobility Disability in Advanced Age

Sedentary individuals are more likely to develop age-related disabilities as they advance in age. The likelihood of this increases coming from a life of inactivity or a setting where only moderate activity is pursued.

Older adults who may have led relatively sedentary lives can be seen as having trouble with simple tasks like dressing and eating. Some may also report as having problems with routines like getting in and out of bed, walking, or other problems that impact personal independence.

A 2014 study followed subjects over a period of ten years where their sedentary behavior, including watching TV, was monitored.

Study results revealed that those who engaged in increased television watching for 5 or more hours every day were an astounding 65% more likely to have a walking disability 10 years down the road.

7 Sitting Undoes the Effects of Exercise

So far, the entire focus of canceling out sedentary behavior is to sit less and move more. More specifically, to engage in some kind of exercise so that muscles and joints are kept in motion and do not get impaired by sitting idle.

In fact, even something as little as sitting down for two hours can erase the health benefits achieved by 20 minutes of exercise.

Your Next Step:
Limit the amount of time you sit. If you find yourself sitting too much then set a timer as a reminder to get up every so often.

Get Your Free Audiobook
Walking for Health and Fitness is proud to introduce:
- the audiobook version, and
- **BONUS 39-page Fitness Movement Guide** of the popular Walking for Health and Fitness eBook.

www.walkingforhealthandfitness.com/whf-ebook-digital-resources

This 2-hour 49-minute audiobook is read by the author and allows you to enjoy great walking information **while… you're out walking!**

II. Basic Training

The basic training section of the book will take you through the physical fitness component of walking.

Not all walking is the same!

- In the *3 Levels of Walking*, I will show you how you can find the walking level that is right for your needs.
- *The Wisdom of Warming Up* will dispel a common misconception about stretching before doing an activity.
- *Supercharge Your Walking* will show you how to apply "STEPS" to improve your walking and show you how to add variations to your walking routine.
- *Cool-Down* will show you how to cool down after a walk.
- I will show you how and why you do *Stretching* after your walk.
- Lastly, *Paths to Fitness* will show you how to get more "bang for your buck".

Chapter 6: 3 Levels of Walking

Level 1: Pleasure Walking
Also described as casual walking as if through a park or mall.

Congratulations! You are ready to join millions of walkers if you can put one foot in front of the other! I call it pleasure walking, because it is what you routinely do every day. This is the "everyday life" type of walking.

You may be asking if this type of walking is of any benefit all. The answer is a resounding YES!

Walking as Little as a Mile a Day at a Comfortable Pace Has Been Shown to:
- Reduce the risks of heart disease
- Increase stamina
- Improve overall health
- Reduce stress
- Improve self-esteem and mood

Think of the recent push to walk 10,000 steps per day.

Pleasure walking has great benefits so, don't miss out on them!

When you are pleasure walking, you can generally walk a mile between 17-24 minutes.

Pleasure walking is a good beginner level, which will build stamina and strength. The focus of this level is your long-term health and an improved quality of life.

How Much Should You Do?
The key will be to focus on consistency rather than intensity. I recommend 30 to 60 minutes of walking per day most days of the week.

You don't have to do the walks all at one time. Several mini-walks are just as effective as one long walk.

Ideas to Get in More Walking Time

- Walk in the morning, at lunchtime, and at dinnertime for at least 10 minutes or more.
- Walk to a local destination instead of driving.
- Park your car a few blocks from your job or other destination.
- Window-shop at the mall.
- Schedule 20-30 minute sessions on a treadmill if you have access on one.

Determine Intensity

Remember, my goal here is to get you out and walking; we don't need to know these numbers in order to enjoy walking, but knowledge is power so with that said, let's see how you can measure intensity.

The Rate of Perceived Exertion

It's how you feel you are exerting yourself on a scale of 1 to 10

- 1 – Sitting on the couch
- 10 – Walking as fast as you can uphill for an hour (OK, that's an exaggeration, but you get the point)

Pleasure walking should feel like a 3-5 on this scale. Only you can determine your rate of perceived exertion.

In Pleasure Walking, it's more important to count miles or minutes walked rather than the intensity of the walk.

Talk Test

An excellent gauge of walking intensity is how difficult it is to carry on a conversation.

When pleasure walking, you should be able to carry on a reasonable conversation while walking.

The Walking Form
- Keep these in mind as you begin to walk:
- Head up and centered
- Shoulders back
- Chest naturally lifted
- Arms low and slightly bent
- Hands loosely cupped
- Abdominals: belly button pulled towards the spine
- Hips loose and natural
- Thighs: natural movement; a link between your hips and lower leg
- Feet: heels strike the ground first
- Breathing and heart rate – Keep breathing smoothly, deeply, and regularly. If breathing in relaxedly, then your heart will beat steadily and rhythmically

The Pleasure Walking Exercise Program!
Get a boost during your next pleasure walk with the Walking for Health and Fitness - **Pleasure Walking Exercise Program!**

www.walkingforhealthandfitness.com/pleasure-walking-exercise-program

Benefits of Affirmations
Developing a positive mindset is an important element of your life success.

Walk and listen to affirmations which are positive statements that describe a desired situation. **"I am healthy, happy, and radiant!"** is an example. It's a positive statement that describes your desire to be a healthy, happy, and radiant person.

Positive affirmations help your internal dialog to create a new vision you have of yourself and your life. The affirmations in this program track are repeated often so the subconscious mind can spring into action.

Level 2: Fitness Walking
Walking at a pace where talking to someone is labored.

What is Fitness Walking?
Fitness walking is a more intense form of walking. In this book, I want to redefine fitness walking as; walking faster and adding bodyweight fitness exercises to supercharge the fitness aspect of walking.

The 2 main goals of this new definition of fitness walking are to increase your heart rate and to build muscle.

3 Ways to Builds a Strong Body and Heart

1. Walk Faster: Older adults capable of walking 2.25 miles per hour or faster consistently lived longer than others within their age group.

Walking speed is a powerful indicator of life expectancy. To increase your walking speed think **STEPS:**
• Shorter quicker strides
• Toes propel you forward
• Engage your core and glutes
• Posture upright
• Swing your arms quickly

2. Walk Uphill: Walking up hills! Does the mere mention of hills send a chill "up" your spine? Love them or hate them they'll still be there so you might as well learn how to walk up hills.

Let's forgo the problems with hills; they're too hard, I'll hurt too much, or I just can't do them. Let's focus on the view from the top and what you can do to reach new heights!

Like any other fitness activity, having more knowledge will get you to easily walk up hills. In no time at all, you will be walking up the tallest, steepest, longest hill on your walking route and not even notice it until you get to the great view at the summit.

You'll conquer hills with some sweat on your brow, a smile on your face, and the satisfaction of knowing that your walking fitness training is paying off!

Benefits of Walking Up Hills
- Increases intensity of your walk
- Quickly improves your fitness
- Increases your heart rate
- Increases the number of calories burned
- Strengthens your quadriceps and hip flexors
- Strengthens your buttocks muscles
- Shapes your entire lower body

How to Efficiently and Easily Walk Up Hills
- Lean forward slightly
- Feel your hips and buttocks assist your thigh muscle (the feel is important)
- Use a relaxed arm swing (do not exaggerate it)
- Use shorter, quicker strides
- Heart Rate: Check your Heart Rate at the top of a climb

To see how much more intense walking uphill is, check your heart rate at both the bottom and top of the hill

How to Check Your Heart Rate
- Find a hill with little or no car traffic and a smooth surface. Here is my favorite hill walk.
- Find a hill with little or no car traffic and a smooth surface. Here is my favorite hill walk.
- Checking your heart rate periodically during a walk is a great way to monitor your fitness progress.
- Feel your pulse for 15 seconds then multiply that number by 4.

For example, if you count 35 beats in 15 seconds that equals 140 beats per minute. (35 X 4=140 beats per minute)

3. Add Bodyweight Fitness Exercises to Your Walking Routine:
By fitness exercises, I mean bodyweight exercises you can do while out walking... no need for special equipment or a gym. Your body will provide all the resistance you need for a fit, firm, and strong body.

Fitness walking is the perfect low impact way to get fit and stay fit! Because fitness walking is so low-impact on your body, there is little risk of injury.

Add a series of bodyweight fitness exercises to supercharge your fitness level! The best part of your new fitness routine is that you will do it during your walks.

Stop at a safe location along your walking route then stop and perform a set of pushups. Then get up and walk for a few minutes then stop and perform pushups again or any number of other bodyweight exercises.

Health Benefits Include
- Weight loss
- Improved health
- Increased energy
- Improved mood
- Stronger muscles and bones
- Longevity

Fitness walking utilizes the hips, buttocks, lower back, abdominals, and upper body muscles.

When you are Fitness Walking, you can generally walk a mile between 14-16 minutes.

Best Bodyweight Exercises to Do While Walking
- Pushups
- Squats

- Lunges
- Shoulder Planks

Benefits of Bodyweight Exercises
Promotes "Youth Hormones"
An Effective strength training regimen promotes the release of vital "youth" hormones:

- Testosterone (for men)
- Estradiol and Estrogen (for women)

Strength training helps prevent the loss of muscular strength known to accompany aging.

It's Free
When I say "strength training" I don't mean heading to the gym and using stationary machines either. Your body weight is all you need to get these fantastic benefits.

Improves Your Balance and Flexibility
Bodyweight training engages your core muscles and improves strength in your limbs.

More than one-third of persons 65 years of age or older fall each year, and in half of such cases, the falls are recurrent.

Falls are the main cause of morbidity and disability in the elderly.

Variety
You have so many choices of exercises. Change it up every workout to tone your whole body.

Change the locations in which to work out. On a beautiful fall day head to a park and enjoy the leaves changing colors. Hot summer day…get to the beach and workout along the shoreline.

"HIIT" – High-Intensity Interval Training"
The HIIT exercises allow you to activate more muscles during your workouts, burn more calories while you work out, and keep burning calories (and activating your cells' mitochondria) after you're done working out.

Quick and to the Point
Quick sets of bodyweight exercises have been proven to help with weight loss more effectively than long cardio sessions. The results of bodyweight exercises is a lean, fit, strong body.

When Should You Begin Fitness Walking?
As pleasure walking gets easier, you'll know it's time to transition to fitness walking.

You should begin fitness walking when you feel comfortable pleasure walking for at least 30 minutes at a time.

As you begin your walking program, you will get to know your body and how it is responding to the new walking routine.

Remember the expression
"Slow and steady wins the race!"

The Walking for Health and Fitness program has been designed for you to get the most out of walking for the remainder of your life.

Fitness does not "travel" on a straight line up. Some days you will need to back off and take it easy. Only you know your body. Always err on the side of caution.

If you don't feel like fitness walking one day, then don't. Going back to pleasure walking is just great.

If you continue to enjoy walking, then my program has done its job!

How to Transition to Fitness Walking?
The following is an excellent way to transition to fitness walking.
You can break this up in any way you'd like.

Here is a Good Way to Start:
- Within a pleasure walk, you pick up the pace for 5 minutes, slow down for 2 minutes, pick it up again for 5 minutes, slow down for 2 then pick it up again for 5 minutes.
- This would give you 15 minutes of fitness walking (approx. 1 mile)

How Much Should You Do?
Fitness walk 3-5 times per week
- As with pleasure walking, it doesn't have to be done all at one time

Gradually Build Up to this Number
- Begin with 1 day in which you fitness walk
- Again, a fitness walk is considered to be 14-16 minutes to cover a mile.
- One day will eventually become two days, two will become three, and so on, and so on!

How To Determining Intensity
Intensity is the major factor for fitness walking!

You Will Track Intensity Via:
Perceived exertion
- Aim for 6-7 on the scale (again, this is your perceived exertion, so only you can determine this).

Talk Test
- Speaking out loud should be an effort. You can only speak in short sentences.
- If you can carry on a full conversation, pick up the pace!
- If you can't speak at all, slow it down!

Walking Form
- Head up and centered
- Shoulders back
- Chest naturally lifted
- Arms low and slightly bent
- Hands loosely cupped
- Abdominals: belly button pulled towards the spine
- Hips loose and natural
- Thighs: natural movement; a link between your hips and lower leg
- Feet: heels strike the ground first
- Breathing and heart rate: keep breathing smoothly, deeply, and regularly. If breathing in a relaxed manner, then your heart will beat steadily and rhythmically.

Research Shows that Walking
- Reduce stress
- Ward off anxiety and feelings of depression
- Boost self-esteem
- Improve sleep

The Fitness Walking Exercise Program
Learn more about The Fitness Walking Exercise Program which takes fitness walking to a new level.

Let me guide you! Within the 35-minute audio track, you will add bodyweight exercises to your walk and complete a 40-second set every 4 minutes. You will complete 8 sets in 32-minutes with a 3 minute cool down… 35-minutes in total for a great workout.

The Fitness Walking Exercise Program supercharges your workout with the addition of positive affirmations spoken to you throughout the workout.
For more information:
www.walkingforhealthandfitness.com/whf-ebook-digital-resources

Level 3: High-Intensity Walking

In a word… fast! High-intensity walking takes fitness walking to the next level.

It incorporates all the benefits of fitness walking and supercharges the number of calories you burn.

You will be pumping your arms more, exaggerating the hip swing, and your walking form will be as if you are on a high wire.

Talking during high-intensity will be severely limited.

Characteristics of High-Intensity Walking
- Faster pace, talking is difficult
- Covering 1 mile between 10-13 minutes

Health Benefits
- Increase in muscle tone
- Improved athletic performance
- Cardio workout
- Greater calorie burn (1.5-2 times as many as fitness walking)

When Should You Begin High-Intensity Walking?
Please remember: The Walking for Health and Fitness Program is all about you getting the greatest benefit from your walk.
- Advancing to this level **is not required** to maintain great health and fitness.
- Please proceed with caution when transitioning to high-intensity walking.
- You have been doing fitness walks (14-16 minutes per mile) for at least 4-6 weeks.
- You can walk a mile in less than 15:30.

Caution: If you currently walk a mile in 18 minutes, then to suddenly trying to walk one in 13 minutes is going to be very difficult and will lead to injury… this is the exact opposite of what I want for you!

How to Transition into High-Intensity Walking
Here is an excellent way to transition into high-intensity walking:

- You have completed the warm-up routine and walked for at least 5 minutes to get the muscles warm.
- You can break this up in any way you'd like, here is a good way to start:
- Within a fitness walk, pick up the pace to high-intensity for 3 minute, slow down for 3, pick it up again for 2 minutes, slow down for 2, then pick it up again for 3 minutes and continue this pattern for 23 minutes.

How fast you walk is subjective. On a scale of 1-10, you should feel like you are walking an 8+ intensity.
This would give you 15 minutes of high-intensity walking!

Reminder
- Gradually build up to longer intensity walks.
- Begin with 1 day in which you fitness walk.
- Again, a fitness walk is considered to be 14-16 minutes to cover a mile.
- One day will eventually become two days, then three days… etc.
- As with fitness walking, it doesn't have to be done all at one time.

How Much Should You Do?
- High-intensity walking should be used as a "hard day" activity, not an everyday type of walk.
- At this level of fitness, use common sense to determine how often you should do a high-intensity walk.
- Your personal goals for health and fitness will determine how much you should do.

Determining Intensity
- Intensity is the major factor for fitness walking.
- You will track intensity via:
- Perceived exertion
- Aim for 8-10 on the scale (again, this is your perceived exertion, so only you can determine this).
- Talk test
- You should barely be able to speak.
- If you can make small talk…pick up the pace!
- If you can't speak at all…slow it down!

Walking Form
Caution: Do not lengthen your stride!
- The secret is to take more steps per minute.
- Imagine you are walking on a tightrope, one leg directly in front of the other.
- Focus on your feet following your arms; focus on matching your stride to your arms movements…the quicker the arms swing, the quicker your legs will move.
- The form is different from fitness walking.
- The hips will feel somewhat uncomfortable and the stride will feel "forced."
- You may need a few walks to get to feel totally comfortable.
- Concentrate more on form rather than speed when you begin to transition to high-intensity walking. If your form is good, the speed will follow.

How-to: Practice Techniques for High-Intensity Walking
Forward lean:
- Exaggerate the lean forward and back as you walk.
- Now just slight lean forward as you walk to get the feel.
- Gradually speed up.

Back and Abdomen:
• Don't stick out your butt.

Shoulders and Arms:
• Think of your spine as a pole with your body rotating around it. Arms should not swing side to side, just straight back and forth.

Hip Action:
• Hips must be flexible to properly move. Concentrate on back and forth instead of side to side hip movement.

Thigh Action:
• Don't over stride.

Food and Ankle Action:
• Focus on toes forward and landing on your heel.

Your Next Step:
Begin as a pleasure walker! As the Nike commercials use to say…**Just Do It!**

**The Walking for Health and Fitness Complete Program
The easiest way to get in shape and stay in shape!**

Chapter 7: The Wisdom of Warming Up

The Big Mistake Most Athletes Make
Just like trying to start your car on a cold morning, your body must also warm up before you can get the most out of it.

The Purpose of a Warm-up is to:
- Increase blood flow to your muscles
- Loosen muscles, joints, tendons, and ligaments
- Make you move more freely
- Cut risk of injury
- Get the brain engaged

The American College of Sports Medicine considers warming up an essential part of any type of workout.

Warming up is a transition between rest and activity.

Download the Exercise Supplement to this Program:
www.walkingforhealthandfitness.com/whf-ebook-digital-resources

The Perfect Warm-up Routine
Crucial but not complicated!
Perform each movement 5 times. This should take approximately 3-5 minutes. A good warm-up will get your body ready to walk and help prevent injuries.

- Squats
- Lunges
- High Knees
- Calf Raises
- Ankle Circles
- Leg Swing (Hold a chair or wall for support)
- Pelvic Loop (Hip Circles)
- Arm Circles

Description of Each Movement
Squats
- Targets the Quadriceps, Glutes, Adductors, Calves, Hamstrings, Hip Flexors, and Abdominal muscles.
- Begin with your feet shoulder width apart
- Slowly drop your butt down towards the floor. Pause at the bottom of the movement and return to standing position.
- Aim to complete 5 squats.

Lunges
- Targets the glutes in your hips and butt. Hamstrings and Quadriceps in your thighs, Calf muscles, Abdominal muscles, and your back muscles act as stabilizers during this exercise.
- Begin with your feet shoulder width apart. Step forward with your left foot and slowly drop your right knee towards the floor.
- Return to the standing position by pushing off the left leg to propel you back.
- Alternate with each leg.
- Aim to complete 5x each leg.

High Knees
- Alternate raising your knees to parallel.
- Helps you to target and strengthen your inner and outer hip area.
- As your body works to maintain balance on the standing leg during the exercise, you can isometrically tone calf, quadriceps, hamstrings, and buttock muscles on the standing leg.
- Begin with feet shoulder width apart and slowly raise you left knee so that your thigh is parallel to the floor.
- Return to standing position.
- Alternate raising each leg.
- Aim to complete 5x each leg.

Calf Raises
- Calf raises exercise the gastrocnemius, tubialis posterior, and soleus muscles of the lower leg.

- The movement performed is the plantar flexion, a.k.a ankle extensions.
- Begin with feet together then slowly raise you heels off the floor.
- Aim to complete 5x.

Ankle Circles
- Loosens the muscles and tendons in the leg and the joint around the foot.
- Doing ankle circles just a few times per week can help you improve flexibility, range of motion, and can improve overall comfort while walking.
- Slightly raise your right leg in front of you. Slowly rotate your foot in a circular motion. Picture you big toe as a pencil point and draw circles with it. Small ones at first then larger as you warm up.
- Aim to complete 5 circles for each ankle.

Leg Swing (Hold a chair or wall for support)
- Leg swings gently engage your hamstrings, quads and calf muscles
- Slowly swing your leg back and forth for 30 seconds on each leg.

Pelvic Loop (Hip Circles)
- This exercise helps loosen the lower back and hip muscles, strengthens the core and trims the waist.
- This exercise is great for relieving stress and tension and improving flexibility.
- Slowly rotate your hips in a circular motion (think Hula-Hoop).
- Slowly rotate clockwise then counter clockwise for 20-30 seconds.

Arm Circles
- This movement targets the shoulders, triceps, biceps, and back.
- Extend your arms out to the side and slowly rotate them in small circles.
- Slowly rotate clockwise then counter clockwise for 20-30 seconds.

So Frank, No Stretching?
Stretching before your muscles are warm and pliable can lead to strains, pulls, and tears. You will stretch during the cool down period after you have walked.

Your Next Step:
Develop your warm-up routine!
Reminder: do not stretch before warming up!

Download the supplemental file with images and descriptions of each movement:
www.walkingforhealthandfitness.com/whf-ebook-digital-resources

Chapter 8: Supercharge Your Walking

To increase your average walking speed, think **More "S.T.E.P.S"**!

Having this simple mental device to remind you of what you need to do will get you moving quickly with just a little practice.

On Your Next Walk Keep "STEPS" in Mind as You Move Forward.
S — Shorter quicker strides
Turnover rate is the key to quicker walking. The more steps you take per minute, the quicker you will walk. Think of a car's piston pumping up and down quickly. You may think that a longer stride would help you walk faster but this is not the case. Increasing your stride puts your legs in an outstretched position which acts as a break. If you walk with music playing, choose songs with different beats per minute then match your steps to the beat. Shorter is better.

T — Toes propel you forward
Push off of the toes of your back foot, which propels you forward for your next step.

E —Engage your core and glutes
Squeeze your glutes and engage your core to support your spine. Strong core muscles; the abdominal muscles, back muscles, and your butt muscles or gluteus maximus are essential to keeping your balance and walking well

P — Posture
Keep your body straight and your head up. This expands the chest cavity and increases your oxygen intake by more than 30 percent. Also, keep your eyes up ahead to help quicken your pace. Use your peripheral vision to watch where your feet will plant on the ground.

S — Swing your arms quickly
An easy way to quicken your walking speed is to quicken the speed at which your arms swing back and forth. If you focus on your arms, your

legs will naturally follow without the urge to lengthen your stride. Keep your arms bent and swing them back and forth in a quick and compact motion to increase momentum. Your shoulders should be relaxed and down.

During each walk, keep **STEPS** in mind. Pick a point in the distance and consciously apply the STEPS in reaching the point. Keep your focus on each of the 5 aspects of STEPS. Eventually, as your body adjusts to the quicker pace, you will just naturally move faster and with more "pep in your step"!

More Ideas to Increase Your Walking Speed
Here is a list of several activities you can do while walking in order to increase the intensity and calorie burn rate.

Pushups
My absolute favorite activity to boost the intensity of my workout is push-ups.

Some benefits of doing push-ups are that they increase functional strength, enhance your cardiovascular system, increase whole body definition, prevent lower back injuries, and improve your posture.

Swing Your Arms
If you want to go faster, take faster steps and focus on your arm swing. Your legs will follow your arms. Faster arm swing leads to faster leg turnover.

DO NOT INCREASE YOUR STRIDE LENGTH

One good option: bend your arms at 90 degrees and pump from the shoulder, like race walkers do.

Also, swing them naturally, as if you're reaching for your wallet in your back pocket. On the swing forward, your wrist should be near the center of your chest.

The vigorous arm pumping allows for a quicker pace and provides a good workout for your upper body.

Add Interval Training

Research shows that interval training, workouts in which you alternate periods of high-intensity exercise with low-intensity recovery periods, increases your fitness and burns more calories over a short period of time than steady-state cardio, or in plain language, just doing the same thing for your whole workout time.

For example, speed up your walking pace for a minute or two every five minutes. Or alternate one fast mile with two slower miles.

Make an effort to walk as much as possible. Skip elevators and escalators and take the stairs. Leave the car at home if you can walk the mile or two to a friend's house. Walk to work, or at least part of the way.

Shoot for a goal of walking for at least 10,000 steps each day. A pedometer or phone apps are available to track your steps.

Choose Varied Terrains

- Walking on grass or gravel burns more calories than walking on a track.
- Walking on soft sand increases caloric expenditure by almost 50 percent.
- Walk up and down hills to build strength and stamina and burn more calories.
- Combine hill walking with your regular flat-terrain walking as a form of interval training.
- When walking uphill, lean forward slightly, as it's easier on your leg muscles.

Walking downhill can be harder on your body, especially the knees, than walking uphill, and may cause muscle soreness, so slow your pace, keep your knees slightly bent, and take shorter steps.

Try a Walking Stick or Poles.
A walking stick is helpful for balance, especially for older people.

To enhance your upper-body workout, use lightweight, rubber-tipped trekking poles, sold in many sporting goods stores.
This is similar to cross-country skiing without the skis.

When you step forward with the left foot, the right arm with the pole comes forward and is planted on the ground, about even with the heel of the left foot.

This works the muscles of your chest and arms as well as some abdominals while reducing the stress on your knees.

Find the right size poles by testing them in the store: you should be able to grip the pole and keep your forearm about level as you walk. Many poles are now adjustable.

Use Hand Weights, but Carefully
Hand weights can boost your caloric expenditure, but they may alter your arm swing and thus lead to muscle soreness or even injury.

They're generally not recommended for people with high blood pressure or heart disease.

If you want to use them, start with one-pound weights and increase the weight gradually.

The weights shouldn't add up to more than 10 percent of your body weight. Ankle weights are not recommended, as they increase the chance of injury.

Try Backward or "Retro" Walking for a Change of Pace
It is demanding since it's a novel activity for most people.

Even a slow pace (2 mph) provides fairly intense training.

"Retro" walking is also a good option if you're trying to vary your workout on a treadmill or stair-climbing machine. And if you're recovering from a knee injury, it may help.

Be Careful When Going Backward Outdoors.
Choose a smooth surface and keep far away from traffic, trees, potholes and other people that are exercising.

A deserted track is ideal for backward walking.

If possible, work out with a spotter, a forward-walking partner who can keep you from bumping into something and help pace you.

To avoid muscle soreness, start slowly: don't try to walk backward more than a quarter mile the first week.

Caution: elderly exercisers or individuals with balance problems should not retro walk.

Walk Faster
Walk quickly for at least half an hour every day, or one hour four times a week. If you weigh 150 pounds, walking at 3.5 miles an hour on flat terrain burns about 300 calories per hour.

This schedule would burn about 1,100 calories a week.

Studies show that burning 1,000 to 2,000 calories a week in exercise helps protect against heart disease.

Your Next Step:
Add some other form of fitness to your walking routine!

Chapter 9: Cool-Down

The Benefits of Cooling Down
Your cool-down is the transition from activity to inactivity.
You can walk at a slower pace for the last 5 minutes of your walk.

Cool-Down Routine:
- Squats
- Lunges
- High Knees
- Calf Raises
- Ankle Circles
- Leg Swing (Hold a chair or wall for support)
- Pelvic Loop (Hip Circles)
- Arm Circles

The Cool-down routine is the same as the warm-up routine.

Your Next Step:
Develop a cool-down routine, then read the next chapter about stretching.
Post-workout is the best time to stretch as your muscles are warm and
more receptive to stretching at this time.

Chapter 10: Stretching

Stretching is an important part of any walking or general fitness routine, but please remember that stretching for 99% of the population is just to get to the point of moving freely and without discomfort.

Everyone has different flexibility in his or her joints and muscles, so if you can't replicate the stretch that an Olympic gymnast can do, that's quite all right; very few people can.

Just focus on feeling comfortable and loose. If you're just starting out, this may take a while…that OK, it will come with consistency.

Stretching helps maintain flexibility, which is how far you can comfortably move your joints. Without stretching, your tendons shorten and tighten.

Flexibility is key to good walking posture.

Good flexibility makes your moves more graceful, free, and fluid.

Flexibility can correct muscle imbalance.

Walking for Health and Fitness Rules for Stretching:
- Hold each stretch for a slow count of 20-30.
- As you hold, take at least two deep breaths.
- Stretch AFTER your walk as your muscles will be pliable and more receptive to stretching.
- Focus on the muscle you are stretching and how it feels.
- Stretching should NEVER cause pain.
- Stretch to the point of mild tension.
- Always stretch after every walk.
- Pay special attention to muscles that feel tight.

The Walking for Health and Fitness Stretching Routine

The Stretches:
- Stretching Routine
- Neck Stretch
- Shoulder Stretch
- Chest Expansion
- Lower Back Stretch
- Hamstring Stretch
- Quadriceps Stretch
- Calf Stretch
- Cat Stretch
- Kneeling Hip Flexor Stretch
- Butterfly
- Figure 4

Download the Supplemental Exercise Guide at:
www.walkingforhealthandfitness.com/whf-ebook-digital-resources

Neck Stretch
- Slowly rotate your head to the left then the right several times.
- Next, slowly drop your chin down and then lift your head up and back. Do this several times.

Shoulder Stretch
- Extend your right arm out in front of you then use your left hand to grab the outer part of the right elbow and slowly pull it across your body.
- Repeat several times then switch arms.

Chest Expansion
- Clasp your hands behind you back, head up, chest out, slowly move your hands away from your back. Hold for 20-30 seconds.
- You will feel a stretch across the chest.

Lower Back Stretch- Standing
(hyperextension)
- Place your hands on your lower back and slowly arch your back as you look up towards the sky.

*Doing this stretch throughout the day** will help alleviate back tension and prevent lower back tightness which leads to back issues.

Lower Back Stretch – On the Floor (hyperextension)
- Begin on the floor in the pushup position then slowly pick your upper body off the floor.
- When beginning this movement start slow. You will gradually increase your range of motion as you perform this stretch over time

Hamstring Stretch 1
- Lean forward with your chest, with hands on your thigh. Do not "round the back". Hold 20-30 seconds.
- Perform this stretch several times on each leg.

Hamstring Stretch 2
- Gently extend your leg up, hold and bring back down. Repeat several time for each leg.
- For added range of motion, grab hold behind your extended knee and gently pull it towards you.

Quadriceps Stretch
- Lift your heel up behind you towards your butt.
- Grab hold of your foot and gently pull your heel towards your butt.
- Slowly slide the knee back slightly.

Calf Stretch 1
- Step forward and keep the back foot heel firmly planted on the ground.
- Slow lean more forward and feel a stretch in the back leg calf.

Calf Stretch 2
- Begin stretching the same as Calf stretch 1, then bend the knee to give a stretch to the shin and lower part of calf.

Cat Stretch
- From your hands and knees, round your back and drop your head and chin down. Breath and hold the stretch 20-30 seconds.
- Then, arch your back and feel the stretch and hold for 20-30 seconds.

Kneeling Hip Flexor Stretch
The hip flexor is in the front of the thigh.
- Knee on one knee and lean back and hold for 20-30 seconds.
- Repeat on opposite leg.

Butterfly
Stretches the groin muscles.
- Sit with the soles of the feet pressed against each other.
- Wedge your elbows against your knees and push down gently then lean forward slightly.

Figure 4 (sitting)
Stretches the piriformis muscle which is a small muscle located deep in the buttock.

If you have tightness in your either butt cheek then perform this stretch after your walk to relieve this tension.

- From the sitting position, place your right foot atop your left knee.
- Lean forward and feel the stretch in your buttocks

Figure 4 (advanced)
- Lay on your back with your feet flat on the floor.
- Put your right leg across your body and rest it on your left knee.
- Reach behind the left knee and gently pull towards you to feel the stretch in your butt.

Your Next Step:
Develop a stretching routine that you will perform after every walk and cool-down.

If I haven't mentioned it enough, download the Exercise Supplemental Guide so you can see the images along with the descriptions. Also get more great bonus content.

Bookmark this page for future reference as I will post links and exclusive content for readers of this book!

www.walkingforhealthandfitness.com/whf-ebook-digital-resources

Chapter 11: Paths to Fitness

Walking can be done anywhere and anytime. Remember to find walking routes that are easy to get to. The easier you make your walking routine, the more you'll get out and walk.

As you get out walking, you will encounter all types of terrain and places to walk. Here are some things to know about the most common places to walk.

Walking Up Hills Gives You More "Bang for the Buck!"
- Increases intensity of your walk
- Quickly improves your fitness
- Increases your heart rate
- Increases the number of calories burned
- Strengthens your quadriceps and hip flexors
- Strengthens your buttocks muscles
- Requires you to lift your legs higher
- Shapes your entire lower body

How to Efficiently Walk Uphill
- Lean forward slightly.
- Feel your hips and buttocks assist your thigh muscle (the feel is important).
- Use a relaxed arm swing (do not exaggerate it).
- Use SHORTER, quicker strides.
- Check your Heart Rate at the top of a climb.
- To see how much more intense walking uphill is, check your heart rate at both the bottom and top of the hill.

How to Measure Your Heart Rate:
- Feel your pulse for 15 seconds then multiply that number by 4.
- For example, if you count 35 beats in 15 seconds that equals 140 beats per minute (35 X 4=140 beats per minute).

- While walking uphill may be difficult at first, the physical benefits you get from walking hills are tremendous!
- I personally love the psychological lift I get from walking and conquering a challenging hill.
- Fortunately, I live in an area of the country with many, many hills of various grades and lengths. I get a real sense of satisfaction as I walk over one for the first time and every time afterwards!

What Goes Up, Must Come Down!
Word of caution on walking down a hill!

Most walking injuries happen on the downhill walk as your foot strike hits the ground harder because your footfall has that little extra to travel.

Your body leans more forward as your center of gravity is shifted. This puts a greater strain on your knees and quadriceps.

How to Walk Downhill
- Walk relaxed
- Smaller controlled steps
- Develop an easy rhythm and pace; the more you walk downhill, the easier it becomes

Walking on a Track
Track walking is an excellent choice for walking, as many tracks have a softer rubberized surface that is easy on the legs. Since most tracks are at or near schools, they usually have water fountains & bathroom facilities nearby.

Walking on a Track Makes it Easy to Keep Track of Your Distance:
- 1 lap=400 meters
- 4 laps is slightly longer than a mile.

It's easier to walk with a partner on a track than the road, as there is plenty of room to walk next to each other, side by side. This can be dangerous when walking on a road.

If you become tired during the walk, the team benches on each sideline give you a place to rest.

Also, you can usually park your vehicle very close by.

You can add variety to your workout by walking up and down the bleacher steps!

Check with your local high school for times that the general public is allowed to use the facilities during off-hours.

My local high school keeps the lights on until 9 pm during the spring, summer, and fall.

Track Walking Etiquette
- Walk on the outer lanes in a counterclockwise direction.
- Always look both ways when stepping onto a track.
- If someone yells "track," they want to pass, so step aside.
- Never stop in the middle of the track.
- Check over your shoulders before you change lanes.

Walking in the Mall
- A great way to get walking miles in!
- Comfortable temperature year-round
- Safety and security
- Restrooms
- Water fountains
- Benches if you become tired
- Parking is close by
- Many malls offer walking programs that begin before the mall opens

Walking in the Woods
Or what we call hiking!
Walking in the woods is a great fitness activity!

Always take along a good trail map and get familiar with it. Be sure to stick to routes that are within your walking abilities.

Many trail associations have information on the Internet about the trails within their jurisdiction. Also, many fellow hikers post trail reviews, comments, and photos of where they have hiked. Take advantage of this resource.

Basic Hiking Information:
- Know the weather forecast!
- Don't get caught out in a storm unprepared.
- Bring along some basic first aid supplies.
- Bring food and water!
- Consider hiking equipment.
- To hike comfortably, you need a good pair of hiking boots which provide ankle support to prevent a rolled ankle.

Hiking Clothes
I always wear long pants due to the risk of Lyme disease from deer ticks.

While there are many, many types of specialty clothes for hiking, you just need the same clothes you would walk in.

Bug Repellent should always be applied before you step into the woods. I've encountered swarms of mosquitoes, gnats, flies— you name it— while hiking in the woods. But, I've never had this problem on my walks through the streets of my town!

Backpack
Due to the amount of gear you need to carry, a large backpack is a must. A good pack has padded shoulder straps to ease the load on you.

Walking Pole
Not a necessity, but they do help you maintain balance on tough up and downhill sections

Hiking Advantages:
- No cars and noise
- Very few people around you… if any! (Also a disadvantage)
- Fresh air
- Most hiking trails lead to someplace interesting such as an overlook, lake or pond, or interesting natural sites such as cliffs, marshes, and rock formations, among so many other points of interest.

Hiking Disadvantages:
- Uneven terrain
- Very few if any people around: always hike with a partner or at the very least tell someone where you are going and when you are expected back. Have a contact system in place in the event of an emergency. For example, if your contact doesn't hear from you by a certain time then they should take the appropriate actions to locate you ASAP!
- You must take with you many more basic supplies than if you are just walking such as a first aid kit, food, and plenty of water.
- Remember, you could be miles away from any help so you must hope for the best and prepare for the worst.

Walking at the Beach
I love doing this while on vacation at the Jersey shore!

- Walk along the edge of the shoreline where the sand is wet and more packed as walking on dry sand is difficult due to your feet sinking into the sand.
- Walking on dry sand is 2 times more difficult than walking on pavement.
- Take caution when walking barefoot. Broken shells or broken glass can cut your feet.
- Take precaution and wear extra sunscreen as there is no shade at the beach.
- Avoid walking during the hottest part of the day 11am-2pm.
- As always, carry water with you.

Walking in the Water
There are two types of water walking:

1. Deep Water
- You are kept afloat by a floatation device.
- Your feet do not touch the bottom.
- You mimic your walking motion while afloat.
- The water adds resistance without the pounding on your body.

2. Shallow Water
- Walking in waist deep (or deeper) water while your feet still touch the bottom.
- The added resistance will keep you from moving quickly, but this is a tough workout.
- Start slowly and gradually increase the amount of time you spend doing this activity.

Your Next Step:
"Spice Up" your walking routine by adding any of the above suggestions.

III. Beyond the Basics

This section of the book will show you how to make the most of the walking experience through other means.

- *Strength Training for Walkers* will improve your fitness level with body-weight and light dumbbell movements.
- *Breathing* will give you a new perspective on this often overlooked but crucial part of fitness.
- *Fixing Minor Injuries* is a basic walker's first aid lesson.
- *Safety First* will keep you alive on the road (no, this is not an overstatement).
- *Rest and Sleep* will help you improve your...rest and sleep!

Chapter 12: Strength Training for Walkers

Why You Need Strength Training
- A complete fitness program contains three important elements:
- Cardiovascular Endurance – Walking
- Flexibility – Stretching
- Strength – Weight Training

Each component enhances the other.

Why Walkers Should Weight Train
- Prevent Injury
- Enhance Performance
- Help Prevent Osteoporosis
- Helps with weight-loss

3 Body Regions
-Lower Body
- Buttocks
- Thighs
- Lower Leg

-Upper Body
- Upper Back
- Chest
- Shoulders
- Arms

-Middle Body
- Abdominals
- Erector Spinae

Weight Training Basics

For our purpose, we just need some very basic equipment. This is not required as most exercises can be accomplished with your body weight.

- Simple dumbbells
- Aerobic step: not required but helpful
- Exercise mat
- Chair

Walking for Health and Fitness Rules of Weight Training

- Rest 30-90 seconds between exercises
- Breathe: exhale as you perform the exercise, inhale as you release the lift
- Lift slowly
- Use proper amount of weight
- Use proper form

Strength Routine:

- Lunge
- Calf Raise
- Pullover
- Push-ups
- Planks
- Front Shoulder Raise
- Back Shoulder Fly
- Bicep curl
- Kickbacks
- Superman Back Exercise
- Dead Bugs
- Pelvic Bridges

Work yourself up to being able to perform 10 repetitions. Then add more sets as you get stronger.

Download the Exercise Supplemental Guide

www.walkingforhealthandfitness.com/whf-ebook-digital-resources

3 Lower Body Movements:
Squat
Squats build your leg muscles including: Quadriceps, hamstring, and calf muscles.
- Hold the dumbbells close to the front of your body.
- Squat down slowly then return to the standing position.

Lunge
Targeted muscles include: Glutes, hamstrings, quadriceps, calf muscles, and abdominal muscles.
- Step forward with one leg and drop the back knee down to the ground.
- Push off front leg to return.

Back muscles work as stabilizers during this exercise.

Calf Raise
- Holding a weight in one hand do one leg at a time.
- Place your feet on the edge of a curb or step.
- Drop the heel down below your toes then raise up.

Review: 3 Lower Body Movements
- Squat
- Lunge
- Calf Raise

Perform each for 10 repetitions.
Gradually build up to 3 sets of 10 reps.

Upper Body Movements:
- Perform each lift slowly.
- Work up to completing
- Complete 10 repetitions for each movement.
- Add more sets to your routine as you get stronger.

Shoulder Press:
Targets the Deltoids, triceps, trapezius, and upper chest muscles.
- Start with the dumbbells at your shoulders
- "Press" them up above your head.

Front Shoulder Raise
Targets the Anterior Deltoid muscles.
- Start with the weights down in front of you.
- Slowly raise one arm so the weight is at eyelevel.
- Slowly lower and repeat.

Back Shoulder Raise (Flyes)
Target the posterior aspects of the shoulder muscles.
- Start with the weight in front of you as you bend slowly at the waist.
- Raise the weights to the side. Lower the weight and repeat.

Bicep Curls
Targets the bicep muscle.
- Start with weights at your side. Pull the weight up by bending at the elbow.
- Squeeze the bicep at the "top" of the lift.
- Alternate each arm.

Tricep Kickbacks
Targets the tricep muscle and rear deltoid.
- Place your right foot forward, bend at the waist, and use your right arm to brace yourself.
- The left arm up bends at the elbow to nearly 90-degrees then lift the weight back.
- Repeat with right arm.

Review: 5 Upper Body Movements:
- Shoulder Press
- Front Shoulder Raise
- Back Shoulder Raise (Flyes)
- Bicep Curls
- Tricep Kickbacks

Perform each for 10 repetitions.
Gradually build up to 3 sets of 10 reps.

Floor Movements:
- Perform each lift slowly.
- Work up to completing 10 repetitions for each movement.
- Add more sets to your routine as you get stronger.

Push-ups
Targets the chest muscles, shoulders, triceps, and abdominals.
- Focus on keeping your body in a straight alignment and your core muscles engaged.
- Place your hands under your body just below your shoulders and push yourself up off the floor.

Planks
Targets the abdominal muscles, glutes, and hamstrings. Supports proper posture and improves balance.
- Place your arms under your body and with elbows bent, raise your whole body off the floor.
- Keep your back and leg straight. Hold this position for 20-30 seconds.
- Work up to holding the plank for 1 minute or more.

Dumbbell Front Pullover
Targets the chest, latissimus dorsi, and tricep muscles.
- Hold a weight above your head
- Slowly lower it behind your head then return it to the start position above your head.

Bird Dog Back Exercise

Improves balance and coordination, making it easier to keep the spine stable for everyday movements such as walking, running, dancing, and carrying a child.

- Alternate lifting and stretching out away from your core the opposite arm and leg.
- Alternate each side.

Dead Bugs

Help Improve your balance, stability, and can help manage lower back pain.

Start Position: Lay on floor, knees up at 90 degrees, arms up towards ceiling.

- Left arm back, right leg drops down heel touch to touch the floor.
- Return to start position.
- Repeat with opposite arm/leg -Right arm back, left leg drops down heel touches the floor.

Pelvic Bridges

Targets the gluteal muscles which make up the buttocks. Also works your core muscles which include the rectus abdominus, erector spinae, hamstrings, and adductors.

- Lay down, feet flat on the floor, heels close to your butt.
- Slowly lift your butt off the floor and keep your body straight from your chest and down through your legs.

Crunches: The Basics

Crunches improve your balance by strengthening your core muscles. Strong core muscles improve posture which helps you function efficiently in everyday life and sports. A healthy posture helps prevent lower back pain and muscle injury.

- Begin with your heels close to your butt, arms crossed at the chest.
- Squeeze your core as you lift upper body from the floor.

Crunches: Variation 1
- Reach across your body and touch the outer part of the opposite knee.
- You should feel no tension in your neck.
- Return to start point and repeat.
- Build up the number of crunches you can complete over time.

Crunches: Variation 2
Start with your feet flat on the floor then lift and move your legs towards your head as your head lifts towards our knees

Build up the number of crunches you can complete over time.

Review: 7 Floor Exercises
- Pushups
- Planks
- Dumbbell Front Pullover
- Bird Dog Back Exercise
- Dead But
- Pelvic Bridge
- Crunches

Perform each for 10 repetitions.
Gradually build up to 3 sets of 10 reps.

Benefits of Logging and Tracking Your Strength Workout
Strength workouts supplement your walks and have incredible benefits that will make you a better walker.

Log your workouts by noting how many pushups or sit ups you are able to do comfortably, and go from there. Are you able to add on two more pushups after a week? Plank for 10 or 20 more seconds?

Regularly Tracking Your Workout Progress is a Must for Several Reasons:
- Makes it more likely to reach and surpass your goal.
- Allows you to be more efficient in your time and workouts.
- Lends accountability to yourself and your goals.
- Allows for easier modifications and shows when and where changes need to be made.
- Can be motivating and reinforcing to remind you why you are doing what you are doing.
- Helps to drive the focus and direction of your programming.
- Keeps you committed to your plan.
- You see your progress!

Your Next Step:
Develop a strength training routine and keep a log of your routine and progress. Keep it simple at first then, as you get stronger, just add more elements to your routine.

*Included in the ***Walking for Health and Fitness Complete Program*** is a strength training how-to videos and training log to assist you in keeping track of your strength progress.

Chapter 13: Breathing

The act of walking is as natural as breathing. Breathing is something we can control and regulate. It is a useful tool for achieving a relaxed and clear state of mind.

I will show you how proper breathing while walking will help you gain the full benefits of walking.

In order to breathe properly, you need to breathe deeply into your abdomen, not just your chest. Your belly should expand as you take a breath in which allows your lungs to fill up to their capacity.

If you have not been breathing this deliberately in the past, it may feel like an effort. Stay with it as your body will quickly "relearn" how to properly breathe.

Breathing exercises should be deep, slow, rhythmic, and through the nose, not through the mouth. The most important part of deep breathing is to regulate your breaths.

I use an odd number pattern to my breathing routine.

Walking and Breathing:
When we use the Odd Number Breathing Cycle, the cycle alternates the start point (or foot we land on) with each cycle of breathing.

Odd Number Breathing Pattern:
• Begin by exhaling from your mouth for a count of 3.
• Then, inhale through the nose, thereby expanding the belly for a count of 4.
• The cycle is a 7 count (an odd number).
• Adjust the pattern as you see fit, but always use an odd number with the inhale 1 count more than the exhale.

Going forward, if you need to shorten the count— especially if breathing gets heavier with more exertion— just change to a 5 count; 2 counts exhale, 3 counts inhale.

Deep Breathing Exercise to Relax:
- Begin by exhaling from your mouth for a count of 3 to expel all the air from your lungs.
- Then, inhale through the nose, thereby expanding the belly for a count of 4.
- Hold your breath in for a count of 7.
- Exhale for a count of 3
- Repeat the pattern

Schedule your deep breathing exercise just as you would schedule important business appointments. Set aside a minimum of two 5-minute segments of time every day to just sit and deep breathe using the Odd Number Breathing Pattern.

Your Next Step:
Begin using the Odd Number Breathing Pattern on your next walk. Start slowly and do it for a few minutes at a time.

As you gain walking experience, you will find yourself effortlessly slipping into this breathing pattern.

Also, set aside time each day to sit and do the deep breathing exercise.

Chapter 14: Fixing Minor Injuries

By choosing walking over other forms of exercise, you have embarked on a journey that is physically and psychologically beneficial. Congratulations!

Walkers have fewer injuries than just about any other fitness group.

Also, many people turn to walking as a way to recover from injuries suffered in other activities.

But we walkers will have some minor issues from time to time so let's learn how to minimize our pain, downtime and recovery time.

The most common pain issue is muscle soreness associated with exercise. This is known as **Delayed Onset Muscle Soreness or DOMS.**

DOMS Treatment:
- Ice
- Rest
- Anti-inflammatory medication
- Massage
- Heat
- Stretching

Other Common Injuries
Nail Problems: Long toenails lead to hitting the front of your shoe causing pain. Get into the habit of cutting and trimming your toenails weekly.

Blisters: Caused by friction and irritation from something rubbing against the foot. Proper shoe fit and quality socks are a must to prevent blisters.

Blister Treatment:
- Lubricate and coat the skin on your feet with petroleum jelly.
- Leave them alone if they don't interfere with walking.
- If they balloon up, then cover them with moleskin or bandages.
- If you must drain them, use a sterilized pin to poke a hole at the bottom edge of the blister. Allow the fluid to drain then treat with an antibiotic cream (Neosporin) and bandage.

Callus: An area of the skin that has become hard which is caused by friction. A callus builds up over time.

Corns: Bumps that crop up all over your feet usually caused by wearing tight, narrow shoes.

Corn Treatment:
- Get rid of the offending shoes will greatly reduce and in some cases eliminate the problem.
- Gently rub your corns with an emery board to decrease the surface area.
- Use a pumice stone for the same purpose.

Bunions: A bony, painful hump at the base of the big toe. Bunions typically start to form in early adulthood as they are hereditary. Tight shoes, especially high heels, push the foot bone into an unnatural shape over time.

Bunion Treatment: Two Types:
-Nonsurgical:
- Reduce the pressure on the toe
- Wear roomy shoes with a big toe box
- Use bunion pads, arch supports, or orthotics (custom made)
- Use protective padding to reduce friction
- Take nonprescription medicine to reduce pain and swelling
- Take a prescription anti-inflammatory (NSAIDs)
- Use ice to relieve pain

-Surgical:
- There are different types of surgical solutions
- Check with your medical doctor to find the right one for you

Neuromas: A bundle of exposed nerve endings characterized by a lack of swelling and the feeling of pain when you are not walking. Again, a tight fitting shoe, which constricts the natural movement of the feet and toes put more pressure on the nerves of the foot.

Neuroma Treatment:
- Ice rubbed over the affected area
- A pad directly behind a neuroma may help ease the pressure
- If the symptoms persist, get to a podiatrist, wear special shoes, and get a Cortisone injection

Plantar Fasciitis: Inflammation of the tough fibrous band of tissue that runs the length of the bottom of your foot. You will feel pain after you walk, not necessarily while you walk. The first few steps out of bed in the morning are painful!

-Causes:
- Over-training
- Misalignment of the foot
- Walking on hard surfaces
- Doing lots of hills
- Putting undue stress on tight hamstrings and calf muscles

-Treatment:
- Plantar Fasciitis responds well to ice and elevation, so immediately after walking, rub a small block of ice along the affected area
- Freeze a water-filled paper cup, then trim the sides to expose the ice. Rub on the hurt area. Also, put your feet in a bucket of ice water
- After ice, prop your feet up (elevate)
- Foot massage
- Over the counter anti-inflammatory

Prevention:
- Keep hamstrings and calf muscles loose
- Stay off hard surfaces (walk on a track, dirt path, or grassy area)
- Avoid hills
- Cross train with non-weight-bearing activities such as cycling and swimming
- Yoga exercises to help keep the body loose

Shin Splints: A catchall term for shin pain and pain in the lower leg due to inflammation of the muscle or tendons.

-Causes:
- Overtraining (walking too much too soon or too often) places stress on the legs during walking and leads to swelling, tearing, and inflammation of the surrounding muscles.
- This is why a gradual buildup of mileage is recommended.

-Prevention:
- Strengthen your shin muscles so that they are in balance with your calf muscles.
- Replace walking shoes often as they lose their cushioning.
- Make sure your shoes fit properly.

-Treatment:
- Some people use ice to help reduce inflammation.
- Other use heat around the shin and calf to help loosen tight muscles.

Lower Back Pain: Typically caused by poor posture and out of balance muscles.

-Causes:
- Muscle of ligament strain (overuse)
- Poor posture
- Bulging or ruptured disks
- Arthritis

- Skeletal irregularities
- Osteoporosis

-Treatment:
- In the first 24 hours, ice the affected area.
- 15 minutes of ice on the back every hour on the hour for 3-4 treatments
- After 24 hours, apply moist heat.
- Heating pad with a moist cloth or thin sponge works great
- Gentle stretching after moist heat

-Prevention:
- Good posture
- Good flexibility
- Don't rush to walk beyond your fitness level... slow and steady wins the race

Rolled Ankle: Caused by stepping awkwardly and stepping on an uneven surface or object.

-Treatment:
- The RICE Method
- Rest, Ice, Compression, and Elevation
- Compression means wrapping the ankle tightly with an ACE bandage.
- In the first 24 hours, ice the affected area.
- 15 minutes of ice on the ankle every hour on the hour for 3-4 treatments
- After 24 hours, apply moist heat.
- A heating pad with a moist cloth or thin sponge works great
- Gentle stretching after moist heat

-Prevention:
- Strengthen ankles by balancing on one foot for 10-30 seconds, then switch feet and repeat the order several times.
- To stabilize yourself on one leg, your feet and ankle must support and balance your body weight.
- Start slowly and only when there is no more pain.

Your Next Step:
Treat any injury as soon as possible! **Better yet**, stay strong and healthy to prevent any injuries in the first place.

Chapter 15: Safety First!

Taking precautions is a must when walking! Let's face it, you will most likely be walking in your neighborhood, and whether urban, suburban, or rural, a good deal of time will be spent on or very near a road.

Be alert while walking at night, and walking in un-crowded, isolated areas.

Other safety concerns will be weather-related: heat, cold, ice, snow, wind, and rain.

21 Walking Safety Tips
Nearly 6000 pedestrians were killed in 2017! Let me repeat that, nearly 6000 pedestrians were killed in 2017 which continued a steadily increasing trend of pedestrian deaths.

Don't become a statistic!

Commit to Following These 21 Walking Safety Tips.
More and more, both drivers and pedestrians are distracted. Distractions are the number three cause of pedestrian fatalities behind speeding and failure to yield which are the two leading causes of pedestrian fatalities.

Fact: Nearly 70 percent of all pedestrian accidents happen at night.

It's been well-documented that drivers are distracted by their devices leading to a rise in traffic crashes. So, before you head out on your next walk, put these 21 walking safety tips into practice.

Taking precautions is a must when walking. Let's face it, you most likely will be walking in your neighborhood and whether urban, suburban, or rural, a good deal of the time you will be on or very near a road.

Also, you may find yourself walking at night, or walking in un-crowded isolated areas.

Let's begin with these 21 pedestrian safety tips and information to make your walking experience a safe, pleasant, and beneficially healthy!

1. **Walk Facing Traffic**: If you remember only one lesson from this book please let it be this, if you walk on the side of the road, **you must face into oncoming traffic**. You need to see what's approaching in order to avoid serious injury.

   If you walk on the side of the road, you must face into oncoming traffic!

2. **Be Seen:** If you remember only two lessons from this book (the first being to face traffic) it's that you must, must, must wear reflective clothing when walking at night. **70% of all pedestrian fatalities happen at night**. It all comes down to reaction time, and drivers can't react to what they don't see. In the daytime, you should always wear bright colored clothing to be seen by drivers.

3. **Crossing Safely at Intersections is Your Responsibility**: Don't assume vehicles will stop! Yes, I know legally, when pedestrians are in a crossway, cars are supposed to stop… the operative words being suppose-to. Let's face it, drivers are distracted, obtuse, clueless, concerned about getting that parking stop just beyond the crosswalk, or any of a hundred different reasons. The crosswalk laws do not mean a thing if you are hurled over the hood of a car because you assumed that you have the right of way. **Be safe, be seen, and be smart**. When crossing a street, make eye contact with the driver of the car. Give them a wave and make sure they see and respond to you. Use the left, right, left rule. Look left, then right, then left again as this is the side of the road cars will be approaching you. Watch for turning vehicles. If a driver cut the corner, you may find yourself under a tire.

4. **Walk Single File on the Road:** While walking side by side is a more natural thing to do, on the road this can only lead to trouble. You are much more exposed to the roadway, and when drivers come around a

blind curve, this could give them and you less reaction time to avoid a collision.

5. **Be "Boring":** What I mean by this is you should just walk in a predictable manner. No sudden swerving out into the roadway, no randomly waving your arms out. See #18 for my cautionary tale.

6. **Walk Defensively:** Don't ever challenge a vehicle or ever assume the drivers know when you have the right of way. Also, err on the side of caution. The very size of a car negates all of your rights as a pedestrian

7. **Always carry Identification and Important Medical Information.**

8. **Don't Walk Alone at Night** (if possible): Working full time, then getting home after the sun sets is common in winter. If you must walk at night please take the following precautions:

-**Wear a reflective vest!** (tip #2) If you remember only two lessons from this book (the first one being to face traffic) then this is number two. A reflective vest will save your life. Think about how many times you have driven at night only to see a pedestrian at the very last moment. Put yourself in the driver's seat…what will make it easier for you to be seen?

-**Carry and use a flashlight or better yet a headlamp.** Headlamps are now a very common household item and are sold at all local hardware and big box stores.

A reflective vest will save your life!

9. **Keep in Contact:** When you are walking alone, let someone know where you'll be walking and when you expect to return, then let that person know that you have returned. This should develop into a habit, and could get you valuable help to you if you miss placing the return call.

10. **Be Alert:** When walking near wooded areas, dense brush, doorways, and courtyards you need to be aware of your surroundings and any possible threats.

11. **Don't Wear Lots of Jewelry or Carry Much Cash**.

12. **Beware of Strangers**: It's unfortunate to even have to write about this but yes, there is always a possibility that you will draw the unwanted attention of the criminal element. Be prepared. Walk in areas that have other walkers, runners, foot traffic, and cars (believe it or not). Acting alert and aware can convince a bad guy that they should move on. For added peace of mind, carry pepper spray or other protection devices.

13. **Protection Devices:** I usually carry a small pepper spray clipped to my belt in case a dog (or human) gets too aggressive for comfort.

14. **Keep Your Earbud Volume Down:** Listening to audiobooks or music while walking is a wonderful way to utilize your time.

-Keep the volume at a level where you can also hear your environment. You need to be aware of cars, kids, dogs, and other factors in order to walk safely. You also thank yourself in years to come that your hearing wasn't blown out while staying in shape.

-A note on headphones: I love to walk and listen to motivational speakers, audiobooks, and music. I listen to some form of audio about 75 percent of the time. My advice is to keep the sound at a reasonable volume so you can also hear what is going on in your surroundings.

15. **Avoid Distracted Walking:** Hang up the phone! Stop talking, stop texting, stop playing games. You will be less likely to anticipate any approaching trouble whether it's drivers, tripping hazards, passing runners, approaching dogs or of more concern, potential criminals that view you as a distracted, easy target.

16. **If You Walk Your Dog:** Keep the leash short so the dog doesn't dart out unexpectedly into traffic or trip a runner or other walkers.

17. **Be Aware of Sun Glare!** In late fall and early spring, during early morning hours, the sun is low on the horizon setting up a situation that on some roadways where drivers are facing east they are looking directly into the sun.

Keep this in mind because during these brief periods of time, drivers:
- Can't see more than a few yards in front of their car.
- Are so focused on the road that they don't see anything else.
- Can't anticipate pedestrians at the curbside ready to cross the road.

I recently had a situation where the sun glare combined with a wet roadway nearly blinded me from above (the sun) and below (the glare from the road). It was so bad that I couldn't see the crossing guard in full neon green reflective gear until I was nearly driving past him. He was standing on the double yellow stripe in the middle of the road. I stopped and cautioned him about the sun glare and for him to be careful as motorists literally can't see him.

18. **Watch and Listen for Runners:** Runners should also follow these rules which put them going in the same direction as you. Listen for footsteps behind you so you are not suddenly startled by a passing runner. This has happened to me a few times and just recently my natural reaction was to lift my arms up in a defensive position which cause me to nearly elbow a woman runner as she passed! She could have avoided this situation by calling out that she was "passing on the right."

19. **Watch and Listen for Bicyclists:** Remember that bike should be riding in the same direction as cars. So, they will be coming at you but, quietly. Pay particular attention while crossing streets as, once again, bikes will be coming at you from the same directions as cars. Think: left, right, left when crossing.

20. **Know Your Walking Limits:** Over-exertion, heat illnesses, frostbite, dehydration, and other serious health issues could happen while overdoing it.

21. **Program 911 Into Your Cellphone:** Also, let someone know your plans. Where you are walking, what time you should return, and make it a habit to contact that person upon your return.

Weather Considerations for Walking
Walking can be done in just about any weather conditions as long as you are prepared and properly dressed. There is a certain kind of satisfaction when I've completed a walk in less than ideal weather conditions. But you must take precautions.

Walking in Hot Weather
Know the heat index which is a result of the combined effects of the temperature and humidity of the air.

For example, if the temperature outside reads 84 degrees, you may think that it is not too warm to walk in, but if the relative humidity is 85%, then the heat index will read 96 degrees.

This could lead to some pretty serious consequences if you are not prepared for this much warmer "real feel" temperature.

Check out the Link Below to the National Weather Service.
www.walkingforhealthandfitness.com/whf-ebook-digital-resources

Helpful Advice:
Acclimatize Yourself to the Warm Weather.
- Begin with short walks as the first hot days arrive
- Gradually increase distance and intensity of your walks
- You must drink lots of water BEFORE, DURING, and AFTER a walk in hot weather
- Carry a water bottle with you and sip from it often in hot weather

- Wear synthetic fabrics that pull moisture away from the body, which allows sweat to evaporate quickly and you to feel more comfortable
- Wear light color clothes to reflect the sun
- Wear sunblock for exposed skin
- Choose a sunblock designed for exercise and sweating
- Wear a hat to protect your scalp
- Wear a good pair of sunglasses
- In extreme heat, back off of your usual pace
- Hot weather can adversely affect your strength and stamina

If You Overheat:
-Heat Cramps
- The seizing up of one or more of your muscles, often the calves
- Often the first sign of heat-related trouble
- If you experience heat cramps
- Stop walking and get to a shaded area
- Gently massage and stretch the affected muscle
- Apply ice if available

-Heat Exhaustion
- Profuse sweating
- Cold clammy skin
- Weak and rapid pulse
- Pale skin
- Dizziness

-If You Experience Heat Exhaustion
- Move into the shade
- Lie down and elevate your feet
- Drink plenty of fluids
- Monitor your pulse & see a doctor for treatment

-Heatstroke
- The most serious of the heat-related illnesses

- You stop perspiring
- Skin is hot and dry to the touch
- Strong but rapid pulse
- Difficulty breathing

-If You Experience Heatstroke
- Get into shade
- Remove as much clothing as possible
- Cool down as quickly as possible
- Water
- Fan
- Air conditioning
- Ice packs
- Wrap yourself in cold wet sheets
- Seek immediate medical attention… meaning – **GET TO A HOSPITAL!**

Hot weather does not have to put an end to your walking routine.

Slowly acclimate yourself to the hot weather, drink plenty of fluids, back off your normal pace for the first few walks in the heat, cover your head from the sun, and in a short amount of time you will be walking your normal routine!

Walking in Cold Weather
Wind and cold together make up wind chill. Know the air temperature and wind chill index before going out to walk.

The key is to dress as if it is 10-degrees warmer than the wind chill temperature.

32-degree weather with a 10 mile per hour wind speed will make it feel like 23 degrees.

Beware of Wind Chill Temperatures
You must take the 9-degree difference between the air temperature reading and the wind chill temperature into account when dressing for the cold.

If you take my advice **BUT** dress 10-degrees warmer than **ONLY** the air temperature (32 degrees), in reality, you would be 19 degrees underdressed (wind chill temperature 23 degrees).

This is the difference between walking comfortably and being miserable.

National Weather Service Wind Chill Calculator:
www.walkingforhealthandfitness.com/whf-ebook-digital-resources

Acclimatize Yourself to the Cold Weather
- Begin with short walks as the first cold days arrive. Gradually increase the distance and intensity of your walks.
- You need as much water in winter as in summer. You must drink lots of water BEFORE, DURING, and AFTER a walk in cold weather.
- Carry a water bottle with you and sip from it often in cold weather.
- Keep your head and neck covered.
- 7% percent of body heat is lost to an uncovered head and neck.
- Your head loses the percentage exposed to the elements, typically 7%.
- You will also lose a great deal of heat between your layers of protection and your neck. Remember that heat rises, and that the body heat you generate will escape unless you stop it with a scarf or bandana.
- Wear gloves to keep your hands warm.
- In extreme cold, cover your nose and face.

Dressing in Layers
Dressing in layers will allow you to regulate your body temperature as you can shed or add layers as needed.
Think of your core as your house furnace. As you walk and do fitness movements you raise your core temperature.

When you properly dress in layers, you can easily capture this heat to stay warm or release it in order to cool down before you sweat too much.

Each layer has a specific job and applying each layer properly will allow you to walk longer, be more comfortable, and enjoy the walking experience.

The Base Layer is closest to your skin. The base layer wicks perspiration away from your skin. You warm up, you begin to perspire, and you want to get the moisture away from your skin as quickly as possible. Go with your preferred fabric, either synthetic or wool, something that is comfortable. As moisture is drawn away from the skin it begins to evaporate.

Avoid cotton as it saturates quickly is very slow to dry out. This will cause you to expend more energy to just keep this now moist layer warm.

The Middle Layer or Insulation Layer helps you retain the heat that radiates from your body. Types of shirts include anything from a thin pullover to a very thick sweater or sweatshirt.

In very cold weather, I've also added a short sleeve shirt over my base layer to add to the insulation factor, then I added a sweatshirt or my new favorite, my wool "Irish" sweater. The more layers you have the easier it is to regulate your body temperature as you can take layers off or put more on as needed.

The Outer Layer provides wind and rain protection. This layer prevents the wind from blowing away warmth built up in the insulation layer and also protects from wet weather.

There are many choices for the outer layer. If you do the base and middle layer correctly, then this could be a little as a light windbreaker. Just recently I walked in 25-degree weather with just my waterproof windbreaker as my outer shell. This jacket has no lining, it just keeps the wind out which is its main job.

Caution:
If you feel a cold wind blowing on your core, then you are losing the
warmth that the insulation layer is trying to trap.

Two Other Factors to Consider in Staying Warm

- **Protect the neck:** wearing a scarf or bandana around your neck will
  also trap the heat generated by your body. You can loosen the scarf to
  allow heat to escape and thus easily regulate your body temperature.

- **Protect the head:** lastly, wearing a hat will also help you retain body
  heat and keep you dry in rainy weather. You do lose a majority of heat
  from your head but since your head is generally 7% of your total body
  surface, only 7% of heat is lost through your head.

It was a popular misconception that you lost 40-50% of body heat through
the head. This is not true.

Important Point:
You don't want to overheat. It's uncomfortable to be sweaty in cold
weather and it could be dangerous. If your base layer is damp it will take
more energy to heat that moisture.

Let's Review:
- The base layer is the most important as it moves perspiration away
  from your skin. Synthetic is an ideal fabric.
- The insulation layer traps warmth around you. Several thinner layers
  are better.
- The outer layer is to keep the wind from blowing away the heat built
  up in the insulation layer.

Your Next Step in Staying Warm:
- Make a game plan for walking in cold weather.
- Go through your clothes and determine which garments will be used for your base, insulation, and outer layer.
- Experiment with different combinations of clothing to find out what keeps you most comfortable.
- Take notes during your cold weather walks as to what you wore and how effective it was.

The Cold Weather Balancing Act
You want to stay warm, but **YOU DON'T WANT TO SWEAT!**
- Sweating in cold weather will cool your body and lead to chills.
- Unzip jackets to let warm air escape
- Undo your scarf to allow the trapped warm air to escape and lower your body temperature.

Keep Legs Covered
- Sweatpants
- Tights
- Thermal Underwear

Sunblock for Exposed Skin
- Especially the nose
- Choose a sunblock designed for exercise and sweating
- Wear proper footwear
- Ice grippers may be needed in snowy, icy conditions
- Boots may be needed in snow

Warming up on a cold day is essential to walking (do the warm-up routine)

Medical Conditions Associated with Cold Weather Walking
Beware of frostbite, which is an injury to the body caused by freezing.

Frostbite is most common on exposed skin. Early warning signs are numbness, loss of feeling, or a stinging sensation.

If you experience frostbite, get out of the cold and slowly warm the affected area. **DO NOT RUB** since this can damage the skin

Hypothermia is abnormally low body temperature.
When you are hypothermic, your body loses more heat faster than it can produce it. Walking in cold, rainy weather increases this risk.

Early warning signs include intense shivering, slurred speech, loss of coordination, and fatigue.

If you experience hypothermia, get out of the cold as soon as possible. Remove wet clothing. This includes clothing that is damp from sweat. Cover up with a blanket and put a hat on. Drink warm beverages.

DO NOT APPLY DIRECT HEAT!

Seek medical attention as soon as possible!

Walking and Climate Factors

Walking on Ice and Snow
- Walking during a light snow shower is one of my most pleasurable walking experiences. The world is quiet, cars are nearly non-existent, and the world is all mine!
- Walking on hard packed, icy, slick, or slushy mess snow is a nuisance at best and dangerous at worst.

If you must walk in ice and snow conditions, take it slow and steady using shorter, quicker strides. Use your arms more to maintain balance.

If the conditions are really awful, use a treadmill or skip walking altogether and do strength training.

Walking in the Rain
In warm weather, walking in the rain is exhilarating! In cold weather, not so much! Wear a waterproof jacket and beware of wind chill temperatures.

Beware of lightning! Do not walk if lightning is present

If you get caught in a lightning storm, head for shelter ASAP. Crouch low touching the ground with only your feet to minimize contact. If possible, get into a car. Also, avoid bodies of water.

Walking in the Wind
You must know the wind chill factor before heading out into the elements. Wear a windbreaker and a hat. Beware of flying debris. If tree limbs are fall all around you…get indoors ASAP

Your Next Step:
Reread this chapter! It's that important!

I'll say it again, reread this chapter it's that important!!!!!

Chapter 16: Rest and Sleep

During sleep, your body is on night shift duty and performs a number of vital functions including:

- Healing damaged cells
- Boosting your immune system
- Recovering from the day's activities
- Recharging your heart and cardiovascular system for the next day

We all know that sleep is important, and we've all experienced the feeling of being refreshed after a good night's sleep – and the feeling of fatigue after a bad night's sleep.

Even though we know this, many of us are not getting the quality sleep needed to truly receive the health benefits of sleep.

What Happens if You Don't Get Enough Sleep?

Your body doesn't get a chance to properly recharge. Over time this lack of sleep will lead to:

- Feeling drowsy, irritable or sometimes depressed.
- Struggling to take in new information at work, remembering things or making decisions.
- Craving more unhealthy foods, which could cause weight gain
- Place a tremendous strain on your nervous system and overall health.

It's important to talk to your doctor and ask if a sleep study is right for you.

6 Secrets to Getting to Sleep Faster

- Avoid afternoon caffeine
- Take a hot bath or sauna
- Bring down the lights
- Keep it cool
- Wear socks to bed
- Have a "get to bed" sleep routine

Natural Sleep Aids
- St. John Wort: Treats depression which affects many aspects of sleep
- Tryptophan: An amino acid that can help the brain relax
- Calcium: Helps the brain use the tryptophan to create melatonin
- Magnesium: Works in conjunction with calcium
- Essential Oils for Sleep: Bergamot, Lavender, Sandalwood, Frankincense, and Mandarin oils can be combined to create a useful sleep-inducing blend
- Passion Flower: Has calming and anti-anxiety effects
- Valerian Root: Has relaxing and sedative-like effects

How Much Sleep Do You Need?
The National Sleep Foundation recommends the following amount of sleep for varying age groups:
- Newborns: 14–17 hours
- Infants: 12–15 hours
- Toddlers 11–14 hours
- Preschoolers 10–13 hours
- School-aged children: 9–11 hours
- Teens: 8–10 hours
- Adults: 7–9 hours
- Older adults: 7–8 hours

Your Next Step:
Develop a good sleep routine and make it a priority to get more quality sleep each and every night.

IV. Mindset

We begin the final section of the book by:

- *Making the Mind-Body Connection*! It's all about the endorphins!
- *Ways to Stay Motivated* will assist you in "getting out the door".
- *29 Things to Do While Walking* will give you ideas on how to make your walks more enjoyable. My hope is that the last item on the list truly inspires you!
- You are what you eat so *Nutrition for Walkers* will give you solid nutritional information.
- *Get Out the Door* will help you do just that.
- I end the book with *Conclusion, About the Author*, my *Thank You!*, and lastly where would we all be without *Social Media!*

Chapter 17: The Mind-Body Connection

You have an extraordinary mind. As the poet John Milton writes in Paradise Lost, "The mind is its own place, and in itself can make a heaven of hell and a hell of heaven."

Benefits of Walking
- Reduce stress
- Ward off anxiety and feelings of depression
- Boost self-esteem
- Improve sleep

How does walking do all this?

Endorphins, Endorphins, Endorphins!
The body produces endorphins in response to prolonged, continuous exercise.

So Why is This So Important?
Endorphins are natural pain and stress fighters. Endorphins are brain chemicals known as neurotransmitters, which transmit electrical signals within the nervous system.

Stress and pain are leading factors in the release of endorphins Endorphins interact with the opiate receptors in the brain to reduce the perception of pain.

Endorphins act similarly to drugs such as morphine and codeine **BUT without the addiction or dependence.** So, endorphins are released to decrease the feeling of pain.

The Secretion of Endorphins Leads to:
- Feeling of euphoria
- Modulation of appetite
- The release of sex hormones
- Enhancement of the immune respons

All these benefits just from exercising! And, walking is our exercise of choice!

This sounds so good, I'm going out for a walk!

More on Endorphins
Endorphin release varies among individuals. Foods such as chocolate or chili peppers can enhance the secretion of endorphins.

Other Activities Stimulate Endorphin Secretion:
- Acupuncture
- Massage
- Mediation
- Yoga

The Act of Walking Makes You More Productive
One of the most interesting findings of the past few decades is that an increase in oxygen is always accompanied by an uptick in mental sharpness. Exercise acts directly on the molecular machinery of the brain itself. It increases neurons' creation, survival, and resistance to damage and stress.

From John Medina's Brain Rules:
Exercise improves cognition for two reasons:
Exercise increases oxygen flow into the brain.
Exercise reduces brain-bound free radicals.

Walking Meditation
Walking, combined with mindful breathing, is by far the most practical and easy to implement method of walking meditation.

It has the added benefit of providing exercise for mind and body at the same time!
- Begin by moving slowly, to find a rhythm to your movements and breathing.

- After you hit that sweet spot where movement and breath get into sync, you can move at any pace you want and walk as long as you like.
- Practice the 4-3 Breathing pattern.
- Inhale for 4 steps, exhale for 3 steps .

The goal is not to make it an effort, but to make it effortless and mindless… meaning that your mind is focused only on the activity itself and not the rest of your day, your problems, your work, or your to-do list.

The goal is to be fully present in the activity of rhythmic movement and breathing.

Thich Nhat Hanh, a Buddhist monk, and author of over 100 books on Zen, describes how it works:

> *"Walking on this planet is a joy. Mindful walking allows us to be aware of the pleasure of walking. We can keep our steps slow, relaxed, and calm. There is no rush, no place to get to, no hurry. Mindful walking can release our sorrows and our worries and help bring peace into our body and mind."*

Walking meditation is way for you to combine meditation with exercise.

Fully focus on the activity itself, rather than the outcome.

Don't think about why you're doing it; weight loss, lowering your cholesterol, or bringing those numbers on your annual blood-work down into the normal range.

Just focus on the activity itself and the rhythmic synchronization of movement and breath in the present moment.

If possible, leave the watch at home. If not, set an alarm and walk until it goes off, then return to where you started.

All of us have been aware of the health benefits of walking for a long time.

The practice of moving meditation is now something that you have been made aware of.

Get outside and enjoy its benefits.

Your Next Step:
Make a conscious effort to truly feel the movement of your body and it's connection to your mental wellbeing. Continue doing the Odd-Number Breathing Pattern on each walk.

Have you tried other programs to get in shape; running, boot camp, weight-training, only to fall short of your goals due to injury, lack of motivation, or just the fact that you disliked doing the exercise?

Walk Listen Connect:
www.walkingforhealthandfitness.com/pleasure-walking-exercise-program

Chapter 18: 10 Ways to Stay Motivated

The definition of motivation is the reason you have for acting or behaving in a particular way.

You need to find that one thing to inspire you to walk. Here are several suggestions to help keep you moving. Of course, your reason for walking may not be on this list and that's just great as long as you have a reason, any reason to keep moving!

Have a Goal
Goals give us purpose! In Chapter 3: Goal Setting Made Simple, I outlined a process to set goals. If you have not set your goal yet, then review that chapter and get started on the road to successful walking!

> **"Goals allow you to control the direction of change in your favor"**
> **~Brian Tracy**

Write It Down
Add as much information as you need to "paint" a complete picture of your walking. I'm constantly added elements to my mileage worksheet.

Fill this out each day to monitor your progress. It's a great feeling when you lookback 6 months from now and see, in writing, how far you've come as a walker.

The Journal will keep you honest. Having a blank entry will get you moving.

10 Ways to Stay Motivated
- Create Vision Board*: This will help you visualize your intended results and allow you to see your ideal future!
- As you create the vision board, your creativity will begin to shine through and fire up your imagination as you literally create your future.
- Break your goals down into smaller pieces.
- Treat yourself whenever you have achieved these smaller pieces.
- Share your walking goals with supportive people.
- Keep yourself organized by having a walking routine.
- Keep the big picture in mind.
- Don't worry about what you can't control.
- Seek out positive information.
- Remind yourself why you set your goals.
- Be consistent.

Your Next Step:
Incorporate some or all of the 10 ways to stay motivated into your walking routine.

Watch my YouTube Video Series: **Keys to Staying Motivated**
Link will be on the Resource Page of this book.

Chapter 19: 29 Things to Do While Walking

There are so many things to do while walking! In fact, I've come up with the top 29 things to do while walking. I've done all of them and they've kept me walking, entertained, and in great shape!

It's a funny thing when I tell people I really enjoy walking, they tell me it's so boring. Quite honestly, I don't get that. I've found so many things to do while walking.

Walking quiets my mind and allows me to think deeper with more clarity and to be more creative with solutions to pressing issues that are on my mind.

When I was a runner, I really couldn't let my mind wander because the exertion involved prevented me from really getting deep inside my own head.

Once I began walking and listening to my inner voice, my thoughts really became crystal clear.

I was able to write down (speak into the iPhone notes app.) all I was thinking, and I was problem solving:
- I created workouts for my Cross-Country team
- I created whole lessons for my various classes
- I designed the Prayer/Zen garden in my backyard
- I've prayed for family and friends
- I came up with the idea to create *The Walking for Health and Fitness Program* in order to help people.

So many good things have come into my life since I began walking that I wanted to share these 29 things to do while walking!

Workout: By combining walking and bodyweight fitness movements you can create the ultimate fitness routine. I love doing push-ups, squats, lunges, or planks at various points of my walks.

I add hills to my route when I want a more challenging walk. By combining walking hills and bodyweight fitness, you increase the numbers of calories you burn during each walk.

Thinking/ Brainstorming: What's your most pressing problem? Stuck with a work-related dilemma? Family issues weighing heavy on you? Walking has a soothing effect on the body and the mind.

I've found the time spent walking has given me more time to think and better analyze problems in my life which has resulted in much better solutions!

Recent research led by the University of California, Los Angeles shows that taking a short walk each day can help to keep the brain healthy, supporting the overall resilience of cognitive functioning.

Day Dream: Getting "lost" in our own world helps you explore new ideas, promotes creativity, improves your memory, solve problems, consolidates learning, improve your IQ, and reflection helps aid your development and well-being!

Now tell me, you couldn't use more of all that!

Pray: Alone with your thoughts, is a great time to get outside of your own head and pray.

Walking Meditation: My idea of walking meditation is to easily walk and breath in an "odd number breathing pattern". For example, I breathe in for 4 steps and breath out for 3 steps this gives me an odd number so that you begin on the opposite foot every 7-step cycle. You can add or decrease the number of steps in the cycle but it must be an odd number.

Also, allow yourself to be aware of the cross-pattern movement of your arm and leg swing which is very meditative.

As you practice this breathing pattern, you'll begin to find that you can quickly drop into it at any time and feel a greater connection of your mind and body. Apply this technique and you'll easily "drop in" to a meditative state.

When the miles pass quickly and you finish your walk refreshed you've hit the meditative sweet spot.

Practice Gratitude: While walking, you can simply take a moment to silently acknowledge all that you have. Giving thanks can transform your life. Gratitude opens the door to more relationships, improves physical health, improves psychological health, helps you sleep better, enhances empathy and reduces aggression, and increases mental strength!

WOW, I'm so grateful to be able to get out and walk most days!

Learn Something:
- Learn a new language: Researchers have found that learning ability and memory retention improves because of the extra blood flow that walking brings.
- Learn a new skill: Need to learn sales? Marketing? Leadership?

Listen to Audiobooks: this is an absolutely fantastic way to enjoy a walk, pass the time quickly, and add to your knowledge base. Are you curious about the origins of the Universe? Need a dose of fiction to entertain you?

There is a wide range of audiobooks that focus on business and work issue. Walk your way to that promotion!

Your local library should have audiobooks in digital, or CD formats for you to borrow.

A good audiobook will entice you to keep walking. On so many occasions, I've continued a walk because of a good audiobook; "I'll walk for just one more chapter"!

Write Something: You can voice your ideas into your smartphone. Most smartphones have very good voice-to-text apps that turn your spoken words into text.

Just download the text when you get home, put them into Word or any other program and you're on your way to writing the great American novel or that work email you've been procrastinating!

Listen to Music: Let the terrain of the road dictate your music. Nice pleasant road with no congestion; choose a soft acoustic guitar instrumental. Long steep hill, I listen to Tom Petty's "Climb that Hill"! Heavy city traffic, then get aggressive and play some heavy metal…not to loud, you need to be aware of your surroundings!

Photography: You can easily carry a small camera or use your smartphone.

Take pictures and find common themes such as trees, flowers, cars, roadside debris, pets, interesting yard statues, etc.

Post them on Instagram or Facebook while you walk!

I post something almost every time I walk. Sometimes it's a nice photo of what I've seen while out walking, other times it's a quote or walking advice.

- Follow me on Instagram: *Walking for Health and Fitness*
- Like me on Facebook: *Walking for Health and Fitness Program*

Track Your Mileage: I've tracked my mileage over the past 14 years (I was a runner until a back injury forced me to walk. Now I'm hooked on walking and my back feels great!) and I've mapped out a route that will take me around the perimeter of the United States.

This started years ago as a way to goof on my students and gave me a reason to get out the door when I was less than motivated. The fun part was photoshopping myself along the route. I tell my students, I've run (now walked), the miles, just not in those locations.

Scavenger Hunt: Look out for certain objects. When I walk, I love finding coins on the road...how in the heck does a dime wind up in a small crack in the road far from any houses?

Reconnect with Family and Friends: Make use of your smartphone by plugging in earbuds with mic capability and you can talk to anyone while you are out walking.

Walk the Dog (if you have one, or your neighbor's dog if you don't): What better way to spend a half-hour than with man's best friend exploring the neighborhood. Walking with your dog has the added benefit of reducing feelings of loneliness for you and your dog.

Enjoy the Environment: Just being outdoors in the fresh air gives you a mental boost. Self-esteem is boosted by all outdoor exercise.

Walk with Friends and Loved Ones: Does it get any better than spending quality time with the people you love and want to be with the most? I've always found that my deepest conversations take place while walking.

Walk for Charity: Many 5k road races allow for walkers to line up at the back of the pack and walk the course. You get in a good walk, and they usually take place on roadways that are blocked off to traffic.

Added benefits include cheering crowds and water stops along the way. Everyone needs to be cheered on from time to time! Extra bonus: The event gets your donation!

Have a Destination in Mind: My long walks are to Starbucks or Dunkin Donuts...coffee, snacks, and bathroom! I usually sit and write down the ideas and thoughts I had while walking.

Find your Happy Place: It's that place that is yours alone where you spend time with yourself. Mine is on a rock ledge overlooking the forest near my home. It's secluded, quiet, peaceful, and I meditate there.

Walk in Pleasant and Enjoyable Places: On the beach at the Jersey Shore is one of my favorite places to walk. Also, this past summer, my family and I walked the Marginal Way Walking Trail in Ogunquit Maine.

Find walking routes that are both scenic and less congested. My new favorite is a route I drive to in the neighboring town. The streets are wide and the houses are big so traffic is kept to a minimum.

Discover, Explore, and Learn History: I frequently walk in the Fort Lee Historic Park overlooking the Hudson River. The park includes a Revolutionary War Museum and paved walking paths.

General George Washington's men were surprised by the British and began the Continental Army's retreat through Bergen County. Fitness and history all in one walk!

Window Shopping/Mall Walking: Map out a route that takes you through your town's main shopping streets.

Another great idea is to hit the mall and mall walk! Indoors, comfortable climate, no rain, places to sit and get a beverage and snack. Perfect!

Do Yoga: As you walk, you can perform some basic yoga such as partial sun salutation. Just walk comfortably and breath in slowly and raise your arms out to your sides and up until both palms touch over your head. Exhale as you bring them down to your sides.

To stretch your chest and shoulders, try the following: Interlace your fingers behind you, with palms toward your back, and gently raise both arms while you continue to walk along. Hold for as long as comfortable. Repeat both moves periodically throughout your walk.

Spread Happiness: Over the years I've noticed the more people on the street I wave to, the more waves I get back. It wasn't long before people began waving to me first. I usually wave to any car that gives me a wide pathway to walk. You can tell beforehand when drivers move to their left as they pass you. I always give these drivers a wave of thanks. I figure the good karma coming my way will help me during the times that fast drivers get too close for comfort.

Rehearse a Presentation or Speech: Do you have a big presentation or speech coming up? Rehearse it out-load on the road during your next walk. Say it out loud with all the hand gestures you need to make a bold statement. No need to feel embarrassed, most people will just think you are talking on your cell phone.

Problem Solve: I usually type out on my iPhone Notes app. two or three pressing problems that I need to resolve. I head out the door without thinking about the problems, then I just let my mind wander. I'm always amazed at how often the solutions just appears and usually in the last 10 minutes of the walk.

I then speak into the app to get it down before it's gone. Give this method a try, be open to the process and you'll find yourself solving many of your most pressing problems.

Community Service: Clean up your walking route. Bring some work gloves and a plastic trash bag with you on your next walk and pick up the cans, bottles, and paper you see along the way.

I notice that most people clean up the front of their property but in wooded sections along a road, most towns only send out a cleaning crew once a year if that.

If nothing else, you get to walk along a tidy road the next time you walk that route.

Start a Business: What Frank? How can you possibly start a business while walking?

Well, you're looking at it! I dreamed **(Day Dream)** about owning my own business and the idea for the idea for *Walking for Health and* Fitness came to me while out on a long walk.

During most walks since then, I have used my walking time to come up with ideas **(Brainstorm)** for a blog post and YouTube video topics.

I've listened to audiobooks **(Learn Something)** to get Internet Marketing advice from marketing professionals, dictated ideas **(Write Something)** into my iPhone notes and planned out **(Thinking)** the contents of my Walking for Health and Fitness eBook and program.

I've taken photos **(Photography)** that have shown up on the website, Facebook page, YouTube videos, Instagram, LinkedIn, Twitter, and Pinterest accounts.

I've learned new skills **(Problem Solving)** to overcome a number of Internet marketing issues including, how to set up an email autoresponder, how to shoot video, and how to write for the web.

Lastly, my hope is that this book helps people in need of health and fitness advice **(Spread Happiness)!**

Notice how many of the 29 things to do while walking showed up in creating and running my Walking for Health and Fitness website and program.

Your Next Step:
There are so many things to do while walking! Pick one of the examples from this list and give it a go.

Explore any one of the 29 things to do while walking. Enjoy yourself, enjoy new places, and learn new things. Exercise has never been this easy and fun, you deserve it!

Included in *The Walking for Health and Fitness Complete Program* are audio tracks of instrumental music to allow yourself to calm your mind and create the health, fitness, and reality of your dreams.

The easiest way to get in shape and stay in shape!

Chapter 20: Nutrition for Walkers

In this chapter, you will learn the basics of good nutrition that will enhance your walking experience and your general wellbeing.

I will not go into any specific diet plan such as low carb, high carb, low protein, high protein, the Paleo diet, or other plans.

This is chapter contains information about what you should eat and drink.

Recent studies have shown that weight loss is associated with eating good, quality foods, including a wide variety of fresh fruits and vegetables.

What is a Calorie?
- A calorie is a unit of heat energy
- Heat energy is what fuels your body the same as gasoline fuels your car's engine.
- Calories are provided by fats, carbohydrates, and proteins

Your Body Utilizes Three Calorie Sources
- Carbohydrates
- Protein
- Fats

The Unique Function of Carbohydrates
- Most readily converted into glycogen, the elementary fuel your body uses.
- An efficient form of energy.
- Breaks down quickly.
- Carbohydrates should be a mainstay of your diet (with caution).

A Word of "Carb" Caution
- The type of Carbohydrate will make all the difference in the world to your health.
- 50-70 percent of your calories should come from carbs.

- There are two types of Carbohydrates:
- Complex (eat more of these)
- Simple (eat less of these)

Complex Carbs
- Loaded with nutrition
- Starchy, bready, grainy, foods which also include vegetables and legumes
- The body absorbs them slowly for steady energy
- Fruits and vegetables:
- They are a combination of both complex and simple carbs
- Are healthy because they contain vitamins, minerals, fiber, and water.

Avoid Simple Carbs
- Candy, cake, doughnuts – anything containing large amounts of processed sugar
- Empty useless calories
- Quickly converted to energy but burn out quickly giving you the roller coaster effect
- Lower energy after half an hour

Protein Function
- Backup fuel supply for the body.
- Made up of amino acids which are the building blocks of the cells, muscles, and tissue.
- Meat, poultry, fish, dairy products, legumes, and nuts.
- While muscle tissue is mostly made up of protein, muscles need the energy to build stronger. So, you must also eat complex carbohydrates to build muscle.
- 15-30 percent of your caloric intake should come from protein.

Fat
- Provides energy.
- A must in your diet.
- Fat intake 15-30 percent of your diet.

- Unfortunately, fats are included in too many processed food so most people go over their optimal needs.

Types of Fat
-Saturated Fats:
- The bad fat.
- Raises "bad" LDL cholesterol.
- Fats from steaks, burgers, butter, cheese, and mayonnaise

-Monounsaturated Fats:
- Lower bad cholesterol without affecting your good cholesterol.
- Olive, canola, and peanut oils.
- Polyunsaturated Fats:

-Good Fats!
- Raise the good HDL cholesterol.
- Sunflower, corn, soy, and canola.

So What Does This All Mean?
So, now you know the 3 calorie sources.
Now what?

General Eating Rule:
- Avoid the simple carbs
- Choose more complex carbs
- Fat is good in moderation
- Choose varied sources of protein

Other Nutritional Factors:
If you follow only one piece of advice from this chapter, then please follow my advice on drinking more water!

Hydration: Water, Water, Water
- Make your water bottle your best friend.

- Water cools your body, aids circulation, digestion, and carries the fuel used to power your muscles.
- The body is 60 percent water.
- Just a 2 percent loss is enough to impair your thinking and judgments.
- Alcohol, caffeine, sun, wind, exercise, smoking, and air conditioning are just a few things that can sap your body of water.
- Drink at least 8 - 8oz. glasses per day.
- Other sources that count towards your 8 per day include:
- Milk, juice, sports drinks, and seltzer.
- Limit or avoid drinks that dehydrate the body:
- Alcohol, coffee, tea, and cola.

Fiber
Indigestible parts of the plant

Two Sources:
-Insoluble Fiber
- Absorbs water and increase bulk in your digestive system
- Keeps things moving along!
- Whole grains, beans, fruits, and vegetables

-Soluble Fiber
- Dissolves in water
- Make you feel fuller
- Whole oats, oat bran

A Word of Caution on Fiber
Don't make a sudden, dramatic increase in your fiber intake. This will lead to gassiness, stomach cramps, and diarrhea. Introduce fiber slowly into your diet!

Vitamins and Minerals
- Neither gives you energy, but your body needs them in order to perform all its chemical reactions.

- Your body needs 40 essential vitamins and minerals to perform at its peak.
- Taking a daily multi-vitamin supplement is a good idea.
- Vitamins come from living sources.
- Minerals come from inorganic or dead sources.
- There is no need to overdo it on vitamins and minerals.
- A well-balanced multi-vitamin is essential.

A Word on Caffeine
- A stimulant that can get you going in the morning!
- Too much caffeine causes an increase in heart rate and metabolism.
- It also can inhibit the body's ability to absorb certain nutrients.
- Some studies show some health benefits to drinking caffeine.

My Advice:
Moderation, moderation, moderation.

I enjoy several cups of coffee a day. My favorite walk is to a Starbucks where I sit for about 40 minutes, contemplate the world around me, do some writing, then continue with my walk!

Avoiding Fast & Junk Foods
Let's face it, fast food is tasty and quick and easy to purchase.

Most fast foods and "junk" foods are loaded with extra fat, salt, and calories and contain very little nutritional value. Why? Because fat and salt taste so good and are so cheap to include in the food.

If You Must Buy Fast Food
- Keep it simple.
- Avoid sandwiches or burgers load with special sauce and cheese.
- Never order a "double" anything.
- Skip the chicken or fish (which sound healthier) if they are fried or batter dipped.

- Barbecued chicken or plain salads are good choices, but avoid the extras such as processed meats, cheese, and creamy dressings on the salad.
- Pancakes or pain English muffins (hold the butter), orange juice and low-fat milk are good choices.
- Pizza is a good fast food—70 percent carbs, 30 percent fat.

Junk Food
- Typically produced in the form of packaged snacks needing little or no preparation.
- Have low nutritional value.

How to Break the Junk Food Habit
Use the Five-Ingredient Rule. If a product has more than 5 ingredients on the label, don't buy it.

Break Your Routine
If you find yourself craving junk food at a certain time each day, do something different such as take a walk, or drink water.

Make Healthy Foods Your Treat!
- Keep healthy food on hand and prepared to eat.
- Slice up your fruits and vegetables beforehand.
- Know what foods trigger your cravings.
- Keep them away from you.

Learn More About The Junk Foods You Eat.
Did you know that frozen "grilled chicken" breasts get their "fresh roasted" marks from a machine infused with vegetable oil?

Chew More Times Than You Need To:
- Chew slowly, consciously, and wait until you finish one bite to take another.
- If you chew more, you'll eat less.

Your Next Step:
Evaluate your diet and eating habits. Replace low-quality foods with better quality foods to fuel your body.

At the very least… **DRINK MORE WATER!**

The Walking for Health and Fitness Complete Program
Learn my "Win-Win Diet Strategy and use the Action Planner for a list of complex carbohydrates to include in your diet.

The easiest way to get in shape and stay in shape!

Chapter 21: Get out the Door Checklist

Getting Out the Door
Many athletes, even professionals, say that the hardest part of training is just getting out the door and starting their workout!

Being organized is beneficial to any fitness routine. The less you have to think about, the more you can focus on the workout ahead.

Walking is an easy sport to prepare for, and having this checklist will save you time and effort as you prepare for your walk!

Over time, getting out the door will be automatic, but a reminder of what to bring along with you is always helpful!

Your Next Step:
Develop a routine for getting out the door:
* Have your walking gear at the ready
* Warm-up

Begin Your Walk:
* Walk
* Cool-down
* Stretch

Enhance Your Fitness and Health:
* Incorporate strength training into your routine
* Improve your eating habits
* Drink more water
* Enjoy the process of Walking for Health and Fitness!

The Get Out the Door Checklist:
IMPORTANT! Check weather conditions and plan according to Wind Chill/Real Feel (cold temperatures) or Heat Index (hot temperatures).

Daytime:
- Sneakers/Shoes
- Clothes
- Id
- Wallet/Money
- Keys
- Phone
- Ear-buds/Headphones
- Hat
- Sunglasses
- Pack
- Water
- Snack
- Contact Person
- Camera

Heat:
- Check Heat Index!
- Water
- Hat
- Shorts
- Light top
- Water (Yes again)
- Sunscreen
- Sunglasses

Cold:
- Check Real Feel/Wind Chill
- Dress in layers
- Hat
- Scarf
- Glove
- Boots in snow/slush
- Water (One more time. It's that important)!

Night-Time: (add these items)
- Reflective Vest!
- Headlamp or Flashlight!

Rain: (add these items)
- Waterproof Jacket
- Reflective Vest (Yes, even in the daytime when it's raining)

Reminder #1:
When walking in the street, **ALWAYS FACE ONCOMING TRAFFIC!**

Reminder #2:
ALWAYS wear a reflective vest and walk with a flashlight at night!

Chapter 22: Conclusion

In his 1997 hit song, "World Tonight," Sir Paul McCartney wrote this line, "I go back so far I'm in front of me". The same could be said about walking. It's been around since man first stood upright and we continue doing it to this day.

Workout fads come and go, but walking has always been and always will be with us.

Follow along with the **"Your Next Step"** suggestions at the end of each chapter and you'll see that walking is the easiest way to get into shape and stay in shape.

The walking lifestyle, and by lifestyle I mean all that you can do to improve your health by walking such as:

- A healthy diet and nutritional habits
- Fitness exercises
- The mental side of walking
- The recreational aspects
- Social aspects

Live a healthier and generally happier life by avoiding the major health-related illnesses listed in Chapter 1.

About the Author

I'm a married father of a wonderful young man.

I am currently a teacher and Cross-County coach and have been an athlete my whole life.

I've played baseball, basketball, ran cross country, lifted weights, and ran thousands of miles while tracking my progress in what I call my "virtual run" around the United States.

Over the years I've goofed on my students about this as I have maps of all the states I "ran" through; first beginning in North Jersey and traveling down US Route 1 to Key West, Fl.

For a laugh, I Photoshopped myself at various landmarks within the states I was running through. I ran the miles… just not in those locals… but my students bought the whole running to Key West ruse.

After completing that "journey" I headed west with the idea of running around the perimeter of the United States. As of 7/30/19, I am on Route 2 nearing the border between New York and Vermont having logged 10,145 miles!

BACK PAIN & THE DREADED DIAGNOSIS
During the fall of 2014, I experienced back pain which then traveled down my left leg. So, I began physical therapy and several months later the pain just suddenly disappears.

I began running again and several months later the pain had returned to my back and left leg and also developed a very sore inner right knee. Only this time I was worse and never responded to my return to physical therapy. Age has a way of slowing the recovery time down.

Then the dreaded diagnosis came from my Orthopedic doctor: "Frank, you've got a herniated disk that looks pretty bad. Stop all activity, rest, and go to a Pain Management doctor. I'm hoping I don't have to operate on you!"

Yeah, that got my attention and for 4 months I did… NOTHING!

No PT, no running, no yoga (as even that hurt), sitting hurt, laying down hurt, everything hurt.

Was I depressed? Maybe, maybe not, but I do know for sure that my thinking and outlook on life became a little "pessimistic or muddied" for lack of a better word.

Three Epidurals later and I was pain free! I returned to teaching and coaching in the fall and quite honestly was too busy and a little afraid to do any type of activity.

RECOVERY AND DISCOVERY
During my recovery period, I began to walk and really began to enjoy it. I live in a hilly area of New Jersey and always included hills in my walk to get a good workout in.

I also began listening to podcasts and audiobooks…this was something I never did while running. The faster pace and intensity of running is not conducive to listening to a good book!

I never missed running during my recovery but I really enjoyed walking!

I loved the solitude, the time for reflection, the podcasts, audiobooks, and great music (I'm a 70's classic rock fan).

Once I began full-time walking, two things happened; I quickly began to lose the weight I had gained during my inactivity, and my thinking became much clearer.

I was healthy, happy, and now felt I had a greater purpose in life and that is to share the awesome benefits of walking with everyone!

Since I began exclusively walking, I've not been injured and created the *Walking for Health and Fitness Program,* and *The Pleasure Walking Mind-Body Connection Program*.

Most of the ideas in the eBook and program came during my daily walks as I took notes with my iPhone! The ultimate in multi-tasking!

Good luck on your health and fitness journey and please reach out to me with any questions you may have.

Did You Like This Book?
Let everyone know by posting a review on Amazon.
A link will be on this books resource page.

Follow My Author Page On Amazon:
Frank S. Ring
Receive notices of new book release, blog and video posts.
A link will be on this books resource page.

Questions or Comments:
Have a question you need to be answered or a comment about the contents of the book or any grammar, proofreading, or formatting issues I should clear up for the next version. Please feel free to email me directly:
Frank@walkingforhealthandfitness.com

Thank You for Purchasing this Book!

Congratulations and great job on deciding to make walking your choice of fitness activity!

I wish you all the health, fitness, happiness, and success in the world and all the best with the rest of your Walking for Health and Fitness journey!

Walk on,
Frank Ring

Author: *Walking for Health and Fitness*, & **Fitness Walking and Bodyweight Exercises**, and my latest book, *Walking Inspiration*!

Social Media:

Follow Walking for Health and Fitness and get more information about the many benefits of walking! Also, contribute your story to our social media platforms

 Walking for Health and Fitness Website

 Walking for Health and Fitness Program

 Walking for Health and Fitness

 WalkingManFrank

 Walking for Health and Fitness

 Walking for Health and Fitness

 Walking for Health and Fitness

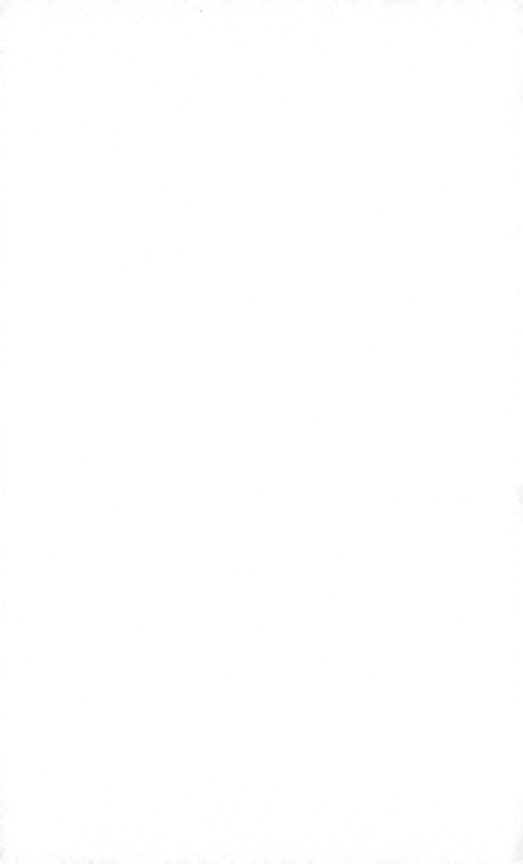

Printed in Great Britain
by Amazon

20472075R00081